Judith von Hall

The Coronavirus Pandemic II

Further Anthroposophical Perspectives

Judith von Halle

THE CORONAVIRUS PANDEMIC

II

Further Anthroposophical Perspectives

Translated by Frank Thomas Smith

These perspectives accompany
"The Coronavirus Pandemic
Anthroposophical Perspectives" (I),
Forest Row 2020

THE CORONAVIRUS PANDEMIC II
FURTHER ANTHROPOSOPHICAL PERSPECTIVES

Originally published in German in 2021 under the title *Die
Coronavirus-Pandemie II: Weitere anthroposophische
Gesichtspunkte* by Verlag für Anthroposophie, Dornach,
Switzerland. Permission to publish this English translation given
by Joseph Morel, representing Judith von Halle: visit their
website at: https://www.v-f-a.ch/

For this English Edition:

Author: Judith von Halle

Translator: Frank Thomas Smith

Cover design: James D. Stewart

Editor: James D. Stewart

For researching this book on-line, see:
https://wn.elib.com/Library/HalleJudithvon/CorPn2_index.html

Anthroposophical Publications
Visit the website at:
https://anthroposophicalpublications.org/

Printed in the United States of America

ISBN: 978-1-948302-35-7 paper
978-1-948302-36-4 eBook

First Printing: May 2022
Anthroposophical Publications

Table of Contents

Foreword 1

Introduction 5

The Fundamental Problems 15

About the Spiritual Character of the Sars-Cov-2 Virus 29

The Consequences of a Covid-19 Infection 47

The Psychical-Spiritual Path of Schooling and Its Effects 57

The Black Lodges and the Soul's Training 71

The Plan of the Black Lodges About Vaccinations 85

Appendix 111

The parable of the unjust steward according to Luke 16, 1-9... 111

About the Author.. 121

Foreword

In this book, the main focus is not on the distressing social developments that have arisen as consequence of the coronavirus pandemic – and for good reason: Although there are already (thankfully) many quality descriptions and articles about this complex of problems and questions, at the same time on the other hand a dangerous knowledge-vacuum has arisen. Therefore in this book I will refrain from elaborating on the problems already made widely visible in favor of this knowledge-vacuum, which will be outlined as an addition to what has already been described in Volume I.

This definitely does not mean that the many undertakings in other fields that are opposed to the divine plan of the Logos, which envisages the development of man as a higher being, are not seen and not recognized as catastrophic.

Such undertakings include, to mention just one of numerous examples, is the debate about compulsory vaccination as well as everything that can be regarded as advantageous or disadvantageous in everyday social life as a result. It will happen, if not today or tomorrow then in a few years, that the spirits opposing the Logos, through the circles of those who wish to serve them on earth, will use scenarios like those of a pandemic to install a general corset of restrictions and regulations that limit the individual human power of decision over one's own being, which will not only include sensory-physical existence, but will also not let the soul-spiritual being of humanity develop, will not allow it to fulfill its spiritual mission in the world. Spiritual totalitarianism is the opposite goal to the impulses of the good.

These developments, or their forerunners today, are not the focus of this study, at least not in detail. For it is meant to deal with a serious "wound," which obviously has neither been discovered nor treated.

In the foreseeable future, an extensive spiritual work of mine will be published by the *Verlag für Anthroposophie*, in which many problems that occupy humanity to an existential degree today and in the near future will be dealt with in detail. So if you miss explanations to these challenges to humanity in this essay, you may consider it as written against the background of what will be presented in that more extensive work.

At the same time, the present essay is related to the hope of being able to draw attention to the fact that it is becoming more and more necessary and urgent for man to gain something in addition to the freedom of decision and self-determination to which he has been entitled since Christ gave it to him, for without it his freedom is of little use: He needs the means to higher consciousness, to spiritual knowledge, in other words: the access of his soul forces to the knowledge of reality, so that on the basis of this knowledge, which enables him to perceive without doubt the actual background and context of the events he encounters on earth, he is in a position to make meaningful decisions which are sustainably constructive for himself and his world.

Gaining higher knowledge is possible for everyone. But it doesn't just fall into your lap. One must be prepared to do something for it, and also to leave something. In order to avoid spiritual totalitarianism one must first know something about what spirituality actually means. And acquiring this knowledge, the most selfless acquisition a person can make, is ultimately at the core of this book.

Berlin, August 15, 2021

Judith von Halle

Introduction

It is surely unusual for the author of a study such as this one to reveal her feelings while writing it; and the reader may consider such private disclosures as inappropriate in such a context.

With this in mind I request your understanding, for I find no other way than to openly express my own feeling of *oppression* as I write this book. Actually, my foremost intention is to work with people who are prepared to enter into a significant spiritual task full speed ahead and without detours, into a work that is focused on the setting of spiritual foundation stones for the soul's future higher development. It is, after all, the *kind of work* which is presently so urgently needed everywhere!

But an obstacle stands in the way of this step. And it is clear that this work cannot begin until that obstacle is removed.

The obstacle is basically that I consider a fruitful spiritual working in community against the background of the heated debates about the "right" way to handle the corona-virus problem to be impossible. For something has entered the anthroposophical movement with "corona" which in form and magnitude has, in my opinion, never been the case before. And what is happening in the anthroposophical movement in this respect is no different than in society as a whole. The populace is deeply divided across all its different social, economic, political, cultural, religious, educational and age groups. And the tendency toward radicalization that becomes apparent when one's own opinion about this subject is expressed compared to that of others, has increased to a worrying extent. One often observes that people have suddenly forgotten their ethical principles and ideals when dealing with others. A moral amnesia seems to have broken out. These developments are catastrophic for people in everyday social life. For a *spiritual* community they mean, in effect, death.

Of course a spiritual, anthroposophical working community should be the appropriate space in which people with different opinions can nevertheless come together, because they know themselves to be united in a higher spirit and strive together for it. If, however, doubts arise among them as to whether the other person truly strives for this spirit because he has a different opinion about the coronavirus question, then such a community is threatened in its very spiritual foundations. Furthermore, in this case a "live" event taking place depends on whether all can agree about how to act in respect to the protection or non-protection from infection. Since I naturally cannot ensure that before every working meeting the participants reach such a formal as well as spiritual agreement among themselves, I see no other possibility than that those people who in the future wish to share a common working group with me reach a basic consensus to accompany the course leader's contribution and participate in the event without "stomach aches," without inner stress.

Originally I wanted what follows to be directed only to the members of the anthroposophical working group of the Free Association for Anthroposophy in Dornach, the Lazarus-John Branch (as well as to those who register for my events) – just as I intended to do with the contents of volume 1. But it's probably an illusion to think that these words will remain in the circle of those for whom they are intended. And I would like very much to avoid a piecemeal way of passing them on, especially in this case. So I have no choice but to attempt to remove the above-mentioned obstacle by means of an official publication.

Although my book is now a public one and therefore accessible to every interested person, I cannot do so except with the background of anthroposophical knowledge of the world and humanity, and the use of certain applicable concepts and basic knowledge. This means that the reader who has not yet come into contact with Anthroposophy may not necessarily find it easy to follow my explanations correctly. This is pointed out here in advance. For this volume also deals with *anthroposophical perspectives.*

Although these words are of course directed at everyone who is open to a somewhat different consideration of outer events, and is basically prepared to accept the reality of a spiritual sovereignty of consciousness as a causally inherent creative force of all things and beings, as well as the importance of the Son of God for the development of the free human being, I am writing mostly for people who, because of being aware of the contents of anthroposophical knowledge, already possess a certain insight into the world and the human being.

But what follows is not only directed to that group of persons because due to their previous knowledge of anthroposophical terminology and contents they will more easily understand, but also because the conditions now seem to be such that among those people who count themselves as members of the anthroposophical movement, it is precisely the "knowing" of certain spiritual facts, or the *handling* of this (mostly read) knowledge, which at an earlier point in time had been provided by a third party (mainly by Rudolf Steiner), does not have to lead directly to enlightenment, but – on the contrary – carries the danger of missing reality by a hair's breadth or even by miles (for which, however, the provider of this spiritual knowledge, Rudolf Steiner, is not to be held in the least responsible).

And here lies the obstacle of which I spoke, not in its essence, but in detail: that within the anthroposophical movement it is precisely because of *knowing* certain statements once made based on spiritual-scientific research that it becomes clear in the present situation what such knowledge is worth if *it alone* is used to judge the present situation, that is, if we confuse certain spiritual- scientific learning with spiritual insight, if we consider what has been acquired by study to be valid spiritual-scientific knowledge. It is apparent in this situation, which has been caused by the coronavirus, that knowing such things can, under certain circumstances, lead in a completely different direction than the one leading to direct, living knowledge of the spiritual facts.

This has – as is evident to me from letters, various internet contributions and articles in anthroposophical journals – led a large (perhaps predominant?) part of anthroposophical oriented circles to adhere to a view of things and events surrounding the coronavirus that not only seems to be almost unprovable, but also makes it clear to me that I am alone out on a limb in my spiritual-scientific consideration of the coronavirus problem, which will be outlined below.

And since the viewpoint that is obviously predominant in large parts of the anthroposophical movement, and which is held with breathless emotion and propagated with an almost missionary zeal, I have little confidence that this book will ultimately lead to anything other than its defamation or the questioning of my spiritual-scientific competence. For a not insignificant number of the letters addressed directly to me contain the wish (or the demand) for agreement by me with their own opinion rather than open questions about understanding of the situation based on spiritual science.

I therefore consider the chance of opening a small door for a different perspective on things through a book like this to be very small. For there is already a certain gate within the anthroposophical movement that is wide open, and through much banging of drums and trumpets apparently many people have already passed through this gate, which opens in only *one* direction.

But I feel obligated, in the best sense of the word, to those who have waited for many months for a statement from me on the present situation and who are really open to considering my answers, although I would like to emphasize that I do not have "the" answer to all your questions! So on one hand there are those whose souls are not yet completely hardened in their conviction, as well as those who have turned to me with the request for an answer, which give me the reason to write and publish this book. And last but not least, as I said, reading this book may help to ensure that the work I actually have in mind can take place in an atmosphere cleared of any ill-feelings, because those who have a strict contradictory view of the sketchy explanations presented here will not want to join (any longer) working groups with me in the future – which is deplorable, but would probably be the only sensible thing in the end.

All these introductory remarks indicate, however, how complicated and deeply regrettable the situation has become.

We are really living in a time in which every individual has fundamental decisions to make – whether they want to or not, whether they are aware of it or not.

However, and this is one of the things that causes me such great distress in writing these thoughts, that at the moment one can actually only identify two major camps of opinion, that tend to be suspicious of each other: for one, that of the "classical," scientifically oriented, essentially un- or-anti-spiritual worldview, the camp in favor of all kinds of exterior protective measures against the coronavirus, who consider it dangerous, and also of those in favor of general regulations and laws and basically supporters of vaccination; and for the other the "alternatives" and otherwise vague definitions or categories, of partly a spiritual, but also a not-at-all spiritual worldview, the position of those who consider the coronavirus harmless, comparable to the influenza virus, the position of supporters of individual freedom of choice in every respect and categorical opponents of vaccination. These two positions accuse each other, sometimes more or less reticently, of fundamental errors and intentions, so that gradually a world appears that seems to be drawn in black and white.

As is indicated in this book, the situation in which we currently find ourselves is not, however, one in which "black" and "white" are as easily distinguishable as many voices today suggest. That this is still widely believed, however, makes it so difficult to untangle the knot, and also to introduce "appealing" evidence for the points to be made, although this in itself is an indication of the nature of the spiritual test we are facing as humanity and as individuals.

I would like to also state now that with this book I have no intention of convincing my readers to change their opinion.

The writing down of the following remarks is not due to a missionary impulse. (In fact, I must admit that I am repelled by writings based on such an impulse.) It is done out of an effort to investigate and deal with the questions brought to me and the cause of the present conditions which have arisen in various areas from the coronavirus problem *by means of anthroposophical spiritual science* – whether a certain opinion is thereby strengthened or weakened.

In a real anthroposophical investigation it cannot be otherwise but that no attention is paid to personal opinions, because it's not a question of personal opinions when we are following the track of spiritual realities. It cannot be understood and operated in any other way than that the personal opinion of the one who undertakes the spiritual-scientific investigation plays such a minor role that – if in the end it proves to be completely insubstantial in relation to reality – the person concerned is prepared to abandon the effort without difficulty.

If otherwise, in such a super-sensible endeavor, one tries (consciously or subconsciously) to confirm his or her own opinion by means of the super-sensible investigation, they may as well not have bothered to undertake such a super-sensory investigation, for it will in fact not be one. Everyone should know this fact who has had first experiences on the path of spiritual training, and is courageous and sincere enough to admit their initial unfortunate errors in this respect.

So it should be clear that this exposition does *not present my personal views* regarding political, economic or external social events. It addresses the *spiritual* challenges which exist for general humanity, and thus within the anthroposophical movement, with regard to the coronavirus issue. It makes no claim to completeness and no claim to complete correctness. But it is the result of a spiritual-scientific investigation carried out to the best of my knowledge and belief and according to the possibilities available to me.

What is therefore explored in this book is considered exclusively according to its spiritual content – according to spiritual-scientific perspectives alone. (This fact may help to answer the question about participation in my events).

The Fundamental Problems of the Present Situation from a Spiritual Viewpoint

From a spiritual point of view *two fundamental* problems appear as the main factors in the present situation, both in regard to the "behavior" of the virus and in regard to our human reaction to the virus itself, as well as to the measures applied or required.

The first of both fundamental problems is the gravest, and it is also the cause of the appearance of the coronavirus in the human sphere: It is *the lack of super-sensible knowledge and therewith the extensive lack of spiritual-scientific insights.*

The *second* fundamental problem is a direct result of the first: *ignoring the actual challenges of the present* by being distracted by external "battlefields."

Of course such things must be worked on. They may not be ignored. The social, economic and political consequences must be addressed. But they can only be wholly and sustainably addressed if the first fundamental problem is addressed, or rather has been addressed. For these battlefields at are provoked and produced by an opposing spirituality in order to fetter the forces of human consciousness which are urgently needed in the field of psychical-spiritual training. The more commitment there is to exterior fields without at the same time an at least equally strong commitment to the psychical-spiritual field, the quicker the efforts of the opposing spirits are realized. The lack of psychical-spiritual awareness was also, as explained in volume I, the cause of the virus's appearance directly in humanity's living space.

The first of the two fundamental problems is therefore a *spiritual knowledge-problem*. And this extends, as stated, to *the nature of the virus* as well as to the spiritual relationships of *the events resulting from the occurrence of the virus*.

That spiritual knowledge of the actual nature or character of the virus will be sought in the natural-scientific world, which currently mostly has an agnostic, purely materialistic view of the world and the human being, is not to be expected. That it will be sought from the anthroposophical side, which has a spiritual view of the world and the human being, is self-evident. But on which foundations are these efforts based?

The majority of articles and appeals which have circulated since the outbreak of the coronavirus and increasingly during the past months (and the related measures mandated by governments) coming from the ambit of the anthroposophical movement rely upon taking Rudolf

Steiner's quotations and transferring them to contemporary events. That they are transfers is of great importance here. For it must be admitted that during Rudolf Steiner's time a coronavirus interacting with humanity in the present way did not exist.

I don't mean to say that it wouldn't be legitimate to include certain statements by Rudolf Steiner about medicine or the efforts of the so-called black lodges (from Rudolf Steiner's time) in the future in judging present-day phenomena. On the contrary. Sound spiritual-scientific knowledge can and should be useful to us! However, we should always be aware of the fact that the transferred statement was not made against the background of contemporary events. Besides, the effort of quoting and coming to one's own conclusions based on these quotations is of course not enough to identify a work as anthroposophical research. Especially since such a procedure can hardly do more than deal with the quotations *selectively*.

Meanwhile lists of all Rudolf Steiner's quotations have been prepared, in which for example the words "black lodges" or "bacilli" appear (the latter word, by the way, being happily transferred to viruses mostly without mentioning it). But as a rule not *all* quotations can be mentioned in one report and handled according to their actual context. *And* – as we realize when reading the numerous articles and essays currently appearing in anthroposophical publications – often people do not *want* to. In mentioning quotations by Rudolf Steiner one proceeds for the most part selectively, consciously or sub-consciously. This is especially noticeable in articles about the *vaccination* question. When one's own standpoint seems supported by Rudolf Steiner's statements apparently critical of vaccination or immunization, the fact that Rudolf Steiner had himself and all his close associates, including children, vaccinated against smallpox, is gladly ignored. Unfortunately, such an approach weakens what might have been essentially justified arguments.

With this example (Rudolf Steiner's smallpox vaccination), it is easy to see how the evaluation of a phenomenon by spiritual-scientific knowledge, as Rudolf Steiner always did when new questions arose, is an individual one, and that spiritual-scientific statements which refer to a specific circumstance can basically not be generalized.

Gathering quotations and building thoughts on them cannot replace what anthroposophy wishes to help people have: the independent ability to gain reliable spiritual knowledge from the phenomena that surrounds us.

Now it's certainly no disgrace today to have not yet achieved such higher capacities of consciousness which could give one the desired clarity about the factual causes and circumstances of the phenomena in question! For to achieve this, a longer path of practice and trial must be completed, and since the conditions for mastering a path to consciousness enlightenment have been available to us for a relatively short time, it is not to be expected otherwise than that many puzzles which are assigned to us today cannot yet be solved in the dreamed of way.

If, however, in the absence of such capabilities (as they are given for now only to certain individuals – for which we may confidently assume the reasons to be the responsibility of wise divine guidance), one thinks to apply spiritual-scientific statements from other times and contexts to the present phenomena, then one should openly and honestly admit that the results arrived at in this way do not necessarily correspond to reality. For if we apply a spiritual-scientific statement to an event that at the point in time when this statement was made was not the object referred to – simply for the reason that the statement was made decades before the event to be analyzed -, then we are doing something which is actually not foreseen in spiritual-scientific procedure: we are *generalizing*.

You can of course be lucky with this procedure and be on target. But it's no less likely that you will miss if you cannot guarantee that the results obtained in this way are supported by a current, independent spiritual-scientific investigation, with autonomous, super-sensible insight.

If an article were to be written in this way, on the coronavirus question for example, and indicated that the author was aware of the possible discrepancy between assertion and reality, the article would be, so to speak, a morally respectable one, morally acceptable and possibly even valuable for further consideration and investigation.

But often the contrary seems to be the case, when you perceive the voices in the anthroposophical movement that mostly stand out. My goodness, how sure they are! So sure that, in order to convince as many souls as possible of their view, do not even shrink from overshooting the mark by using methods that they criticize when used by the "opposition"; for example statistics (often very questionable ones), or by seeking the support of personalities who are far from having an anthroposophical view of humanity or from recognizing the reality of the creating spirit in the material world, or by making assertions which anyone who walks through the world with open eyes can easily refute, and will.

These include claims (which, by the way, are propagated by personalities who – unlike the representatives of the first-mentioned group – claim super- sensory research competence) such as the one that the cause of the many Covid 19 illnesses and even of many deaths, among other things, is to be found in the coronavirus tests and in the wearing of masks, but not in the classical virus infection. After a year and a half of pandemic regulations, when every one of us have often and at diverse opportunities worn a protective breathing mask, we will surely have realized that neither they nor their human companions have become ill or died because of wearing the masks. This by no means implies that wearing a mask does not have an incisive, burdensome social effect or that it can be felt as unpleasant – depending on personal sensibility (people with respiratory illnesses are of course not included). But that a coronavirus infection or even death could be caused by wearing a mask is simply an untenable assertion. Those who make such an assertion should ask themselves where all the people are who have become ill or died from wearing such protective masks, if not in their own ranks. There are professional branches, for example the chemical industry, biochemistry or medicine, in which thousands of people have spent their whole professional lives, decades before the coronavirus outbreak and the introduction of pandemic regulations, day in and day out, ten hours or longer having worn OP-FFP-2 and FFP- 3 masks, and still do.

In all those decades no professional branch has become known for masses of people (or any at all) getting ill or dying from wearing a protective mask. On the contrary. They are called *protective* masks to *protect* the respiratory paths from illness in such risky professions.

It's similar with the assertion about the corona-tests. I have tested myself and have let myself be tested. And just as little as I have become ill or died from wearing an FFFP-2 mask, have I become ill or died of Covid-19 or any other ailment from using the corona tests. The same is true for many close or distant acquaintances. Nor have I been limited in my spiritual working capacity after the corona tests, and I have also not been manipulated or has my consciousness been controlled from outside by nanoparticles or nano-robots supposedly introduced through my nose and throat.

Such assertions do nothing for anthroposophy. Instead they are more apt to disparage not only the anthroposophical movement, but also Anthroposophy as such – and therewith Rudolf Steiner -, and do lasting damage to the impulse that has come into the world to help the psychical- spiritual path of training toward humanity's higher consciousness through the spiritual-scientific approach. Of course, it is not a matter of speaking to a materialistically minded world in a manner compatible with it by representing a worldview which is the opposite of Anthroposophy's, or one not recognizing the spirit at all! Rather by such behavior, by the spreading of untenable, absurd assertions, one undoubtedly drives away a significant number of people from Anthroposophy who are

THE CORONAVIRUS PANDEMIC II

looking for serious spiritual orientation, because they must assume that the teachings of spiritual science and the anthroposophical path of training are similarly absurd and eccentric as some theses coming from the anthroposophical movement on the coronavirus question – as if the anthroposophical impulse did not have enough problems to get through already!

This is also a reason, as mentioned at the beginning, why writing this book so depresses me. That such things must be discussed at all is shattering. And feelings are so heated and thoughts and convictions so gridlocked that I fear I won't be able to make myself understood under these conditions.

For whether within the anthroposophical movement one depends on quotations (like the ones mentioned above about the testing and mask questions) or on one's own super-sensory insights, there is agreement on one point, namely that the "enemy" can be identified and named: the governments that impose unreasonable measures, as well as the representatives of science and the pharmaceutical industry, through whom people are driven to desperation and dependence and through whom a climate of fear is spread. (Whereby one is obviously unaware that by spreading horror stories about wearing the mask being the cause of innumerable sicknesses and deaths, an equally severe climate of fear ensures, yes, even a kind of mass hysteria. As a result of which people are disposed to interpret diverse sensitivities, which they would normally not consider worth worrying about, as the effect of wearing a mask, and are fully alert for any sign that seems to confirm the horror stories. – There are enough true horror stories, sense perceptible as well as super-sensibly perceptible ones! There is no need to invent more – neither on the side of the pharma-industry and the investigators and physicians or politicians dependent on it, or on the side of the alternative movement and especially not the anthroposophical one.)

Having said this, the reader should not assume that I do *not* consider the restriction of democratic basic rights to be an extremely serious matter (although I sometimes do wish that people would show themselves capable of accepting the necessary personal responsibility). Nor should he think that I do *not* consider the attempts at manipulation of journalism and the media that are being made ever-increasingly today to be a fundamental gambit on the part of the opposing spirits. Nor should the reader think that I do not see the terrible social and economic effects. And it is in no way meant or said that an ever stronger anti-spiritual, purely materialistic impulse of thought and will is strongly being exerted by those opposing spirits who are pursuing a goal contrary to the higher development of humanity in a systematic way, largely unchecked.

But if you want to make the effort to unravel the twisted threads a little, you cannot avoid and should not avoid calling the coronavirus an attack of the "anti-spirit-powers" and pointing a finger at the weak point of the argumentation, which does not emphasize the virus itself, but solely events about and around the virus. For what is being said (also by many in the anthroposophical movement) and upon which all subsequent explanations depend, is more or less the following: *If the government, which restricts fundamental rights and makes public health the plaything of materialistic natural science and a predatory capitalistic pharmaceutical industry, holds the virus to be dangerous, then the virus must in reality be harmless.*

But if one examines the interrelationships with spiritual-scientific means of cognition, this conclusion proves to be a "short circuit"! And this short circuit has two serious consequences: The first consequence is that one overlooks or underestimates the actual nature or spiritual quality of the virus. And the second consequence is black and white thinking, with which you look for faults in the outside world, that is, in "the others," which leads to condemning thinking, emotional harshness, tendency to radicalization, suspicion and, finally, to social separation, and even to open aggression toward every fellow human being who merely supports a different opinion. But haven't we then come to exactly where the "counter-spiritual-powers" want us?

And isn't it logical that these counter-spiritual powers – which must feel particularly threatened by people who don't fall for the idea of a materialistic view of the world and of humanity – are not content with deceiving the gullible "masses," but concentrate on the confusion of precisely such people who could become dangerous to their project?

In view of this easily recognizable fact, would it not be possible, especially by members of the anthroposophical movement, to be a little more cautious about the certainty of their own convictions, to periodically self-question and take a dispassionate step back from one's own opinions, in order to become aware of possible errors or "traps" into which one might have fallen?

Wouldn't it be downright catastrophic if the justified efforts of those who are attentive to the super-sensory knowledge of the world and humanity, and who are now engaged in writing articles and newsletters so that humanity may be aware of the influence and plans of the anti-spiritual hierarchies, should fade away like a discordance because of the "short circuit" mentioned above – or if they were even to point people in the wrong direction?

If one is to do justice to a legitimate effort concerning the coronavirus issue, more must be accomplished than conducting a trial based on circumstantial evidence. For (as has already been mentioned many times elsewhere) materialism has meanwhile crept into our way of thinking, and it therefore also threatens anthroposophy in that spiritual-scientific communications are often treated as matter, by making them into objects which we then try to use to confirm our own ideas and convictions, which must then lead to a "materialization" and there with, an "intellectualization" of spiritual science. Should we not therefore – as is practiced in any case on the anthroposophical path of training – take a step back and try, in complete freedom and from one's own point of view, to explore the real context *beyond the threshold* of what seems so evident in the coronavirus question? When we do so, however, it becomes apparent that the assessment that the Sars-CoV-2 virus is no worse than ordinary flu is a horrendous mistake!

This confirmation results from a purely super-sensory view, that is, completely independent of what a more or less materialistic scientific research says about the coronavirus; and independent of what virologists or politicians have to say about it. It results from the purely spiritual viewpoint that the encounter of the human being with the Sars-CoV-2 virus represents a real danger for human development – a danger which obviously has hardly or not at all been recognized until now by both the materialistically thinking and non-materialistically thinking sides.

If someone holds Sars-CoV-2 dangerous from a purely natural scientific standpoint, and if someone else holds Sars-Cov-2 harmless from an alternative or holistic standpoint, neither has recognized the spiritual dimension of Sars-CoV-2 (The latter one has also underestimated the purely physiological effects of a Covid-19 infection and simply refuses to acknowledge the factual and obvious differences in the course of the illnesses and the aftereffects of influenza and Covid-19 infections.)

So if you want to take the bull by the horns and allow the light of knowledge to shine into the confused circumstances and open questions, if you want to represent the spiritual facts to the world in the right way and strongly, you must do so *differently* than by pasting quotations together or by falling back on exaggerated or false assertions.

The strengthening of the anthroposophical standpoint begins with the spiritual-scientific *consideration of the Sars-CoV-2-Virus itself*, for at the present time powerful counter-spirit-powers are at work which intend to hinder the illumination of humanity's consciousness and thereby steal away the seed of inner freedom gained through the Christ deed.

About the Spiritual Character of the Sars-Cov-2 Virus

Regarding my own (aphoristic) contribution here, I would like to add that I consider the whole investigation of the coronavirus question, especially with regard to the "behavior" of the virus, as well as to the effects of vaccination, as an extremely complex area of research, which I do not claim to be able to fathom and evaluate completely! Not only are the highest ranking (so to speak) forces involved that stand opposed to the good divine hierarchies, but it's a case of a "happening in development" – not a finished event that can be investigated and definitively evaluated. Like the virus itself, the entire process with its many sidetracks continues to evolve – dependent upon how the human being behaves relative to himself and the living universal active spirit, as well as his potential for higher consciousness.

In my first volume about the Sars-CoV-2-Virus (*The Coronavirus Pandemic – Anthroposophical Perspectives*, Forest Row 2021 [6]) I wrote that the "nature" of this virus indicated to me that it is the direct result of humanity's spiritual failure in the area of thinking, a result or "metamorphosis" therefore, of the thinking materialism of the past 150 years. Humanity is breathing, along with the Sars-CoV-2-Virus, the manifested results of its own destructive thinking in respect to the spirit and man's higher development. And I tried to point out that this fact is given a particularly dramatic impetus by the fact that the spiritual force, or anti-spiritual force, which is in opposition to the spiritual individuality or the "I" (in contrast to the ego or self) of man, is attempting to take advantage of this event by using those thoughts of humanity which have now become manifest (or material) as the Sars-CoV-2-Virus, as a means of preventing the higher development of man under the leadership of his I.

Conventional science regards the virus as a potential danger coming from without, which causally has nothing to do with human beings and against which the organism must defend itself.

In anthroposophical circles, however, the notion exists, based on certain remarks by Rudolf Steiner, that – simply stated – things coming from outside do not by themselves attack human beings, who bring them on themselves, so to speak, because it is a fact that man, through his spiritual being, is related to everything that exists and is active in the world; so that the notion of an outside and an inside as worlds closed from each other can only have a certain justification on the purely physical-material level, but not with regard to the whole real organism of the human being, which does not only include the physical-material body, but also a spiritual physical body, a life-body, a soul-body, and its spiritual core. Through the latter man encounters what enters into his physical organism on a different level than on the purely physical-material one. And since the spiritual core contains the potency to assess its own events of destiny from prenatal existence, and then implement them in this incarnation, completely different criteria emerge when considering the aspects of health and illness.

If one transfers this thought to infections, one can, as mentioned, arrive at the notion that it is the whole human organism itself that ingests the bacteria or virus into itself and interacts with it in order to finally benefit from the meeting; so that one may not regard the encounter with a pathogen as something from which one has to protect the human being by all possible means. The encounter with certain pathogens is – on the contrary – essential for life in a material body on a material earth. (By the way, scientific circles that are adverse to Anthroposophy come to similar conclusions today, only they do not recognize the leading spirit behind what is happening, namely the actual, the higher human being.) If conventional science is of the opinion that the immune system must be supported by vaccination in its defense against the attacker, then from the anthroposophical point of view this is not accepted as an act of support, for the reasons outlined above. One must fear that by a vaccination one rather takes away the strength from the (spiritually led) human organism to integrate itself independently and autonomously into life on the physical plane.

Now, however, in many circles of the anthroposophical movement this view has become a "sacred cow," an untouchable "Holy Grail" that can never be questioned. Such rigidity must be recognized as fundamentally unrealistic, especially to someone who has experienced the nature of the living universal spirit (see Rudolf Steiner's smallpox vaccination). But precisely now, with respect to the Sars-coV-2-Virus (and doubtless with respect to many other viruses that will emerge in the near future) it must be recognized to super-sensible contemplation as fatal!

One could say that everything that has been previously indicated is still valid. However, due to the fact that the "emergence" of the virus took place under conditions that have never existed in the history of the world until recently, the portents of all parameters suddenly change. And since no serious anthroposophical research has been (or can be) undertaken, basically the same thing happens in large circles of the anthroposophical movement as in conventional scientific circles: Although in anthroposophical circles it is recognized that it is the person who takes the virus in "from outside" instead of being invaded by it, it is nevertheless believed, exactly as in other circles, that the psychical-spiritual human being is *not the cause* of the coronavirus pandemic.

The fact that humanity has been negligent in respect to the I, that it has hardly activated what in anthroposophical terminology is called the "consciousness-soul" or, in the broadest sense, not activated it at all, *although it could have done so long ago* (whereby the sacrificial act and gift of the Christ would have led to its actual purpose and fulfillment), has led to the fact that humanity not only prepares its fate itself – as it already did previously – but that since recently – in contrast to previously – *it does not have the means* to respond to its self-prepared fate in a beneficial way. Because until recently, when man had not yet been negligent in respect to his I, what is sometimes called in the anthroposophical movement the "peripheral" I was responsible and sufficiently so, in responding to a viral pathogen. Up until that point the infectious disease was, so to speak, a vegetative process, which was beyond the human being's consciousness. It was only by means of his physiological reactions, for example fevers, that he could sense that a "higher something" was active in him. Neither could he, his daylight consciousness that is, lead the altercation with the pathogen – *nor did he need to!*

However, due to the fact that in the meantime a serious negligence of the I has occurred, because of which the human being has not deployed his consciousness-soul at a time when he could and should have, but instead has produced overripe, rotten fruits of the comprehension-soul, which have now become manifest on the *physical plane* in the form of the said virus, and the neglect is springing upon him today with brunt force as a *demand*: He would have to be able to respond to the virus – or rather all bodily processes that have taken place in his organism during earlier infections when still under the guidance of his higher I acting from the periphery, and thus unnoticed by his consciousness – *consciously* from *within* his bodily existence! For the neglect consisted in the fact that he made no effort to bring his higher I from the periphery into his inner being in order to let it become active from within. In order to compensate for the danger he created for himself by his neglect, that is, to resist the harmful effect of the Sars-CoV-2 virus and transform it into a form that is useful or at least does not harm him any further, he would now have to be able to conduct those bodily processes self-sufficiently by his higher consciousness, which his wise higher I had conducted before from outside of his body, that is, without his daylight consciousness! So the higher I would have to shift completely into his physical body, awaken completely in his ordinary consciousness down to the bodily processes, or, expressed differently: humanity would have to awaken from its ordinary consciousness to its higher I-consciousness to an extent that would allow it to consciously control its immunization processes – *an impossible task!*

Even if humanity had *not* neglected its consciousness-soul activity during the past 150 years, it would still be far from being in a condition to perform such a conscious act. (Nevertheless, in that case it would not have had something removed, which has now returned in the form of a coronavirus.)

One can visualize what has been described here, but not the enormous dimension of the monstrous "nature," the spirituality or rather "unspirituality" of what underlies the Sars-CoV-2 virus!

In view of this circumstance it is hardly bearable when from many directions of the anthroposophical movement it is proclaimed that the Sars-CoV-2 virus can be classified as harmless, that it is basically indistinguishable from an ordinary flu virus, and there is even spin of a "benign" I of the virus that people should invite in and embrace. And the fact that the "official" side of the anthroposophical movement advocates for protective measures and vaccinations, although they obviously have no knowledge of the contexts presented here, or at least do not say anything about them, cannot be called very hopeful either.

This virus, with its currently known mutations or variants, is only the very weak advance guard of pathogens of much greater caliber. But the origin and the "stowaway" of the Sars-CoV-2 virus are the same as the pathogens that will follow in the future. For if man does not now make an about-face in his attitude towards his own, namely spiritual, nature, if he does not now, because of this event, which is more than just a warning shot, arrange conditions for developing "organs" with which he is able to comprehend reality and thereby engage in completely different behavior, his new neglect will spread exponentially on the physical plane and rush toward it. (And the problem of pathogens, which are in principle uncontrollable by one's own spiritual forces, will not be the only one against which humanity will have to fight, as is already indicated today by climate change and its consequences – as a "minor" example.) It is a pandemic event. It is an event which – because its causal neglect is of a *spiritual*, which means moral nature – affects *all* human beings, also those who may be less responsible for the spiritual neglect. They will also have to suffer under this kind of plague. What humanity will then have also accomplished is to pull the basic needs for life out from under the bearers of hope sent to it by the spiritual world as impulse for the good. And within the raging storms against the spirit in which humanity finds itself, it would have thrown away the torch which could have given it some orientation in the darkness.

I am aware that these lines weigh heavily. I am aware that nobody likes to read such "messages." I am aware that one prefers to read and agree with viewpoints that present our current situation in a more hopeful light, which perhaps even give the "all-clear," especially when they are sprinkled with all kinds of conclusive quotations from Rudolf Steiner – and not infrequently (this should be disconcerting) with all kinds of confirming contributions coming from personalities who otherwise have not the slightest interest in anthroposophical knowledge of man and the world.

Yes, I am aware that the description of these gloomy conditions and prospects is not what the soul wants to hear. But if a fire flares up in the room no one will want to lie in bed and pretend not to know about it, hoping that in that way the flames will disappear. He would, on the contrary, certainly jump up and try to extinguish the fire. And if he had been asleep during the burgeoning fire, he would certainly be glad later that his neighbor, who noticed the fire, had woken him up. And he would certainly not blame having woken up for the fact that his bedroom is no longer as cozy as it was before the fire.

If with this in mind one looks back once again at the method outlined above, which is so frequently used today, namely to draw conclusions regarding current events based on Rudolf Steiner's spiritual-scientific research, then adds to this mental construction one's own ideas that seem to fit on top, and in this way judges the situation and subsequently recommends a certain behavior to others. From this one can recognize how "diabolical" the coronavirus (or rather the counter-spirit working through it) operates, even without the path of an infection. By using this method one runs the risk of confusing true from false. Everything fits together conclusively. Everything seems suddenly crystal clear! Euphoria percolates. One wishes to spread what is so clearly evident in the form of articles, newsletters and lectures in order to guide others to enlightenment as well. And it seldom happens that one wonders why suddenly people share or approve one's own convictions who may not want to know the slightest thing about Anthroposophy (in whose center Christ stands) and the ideals to which the anthroposophical spiritual student strives. But the conviction that one has clearly localized the evil and, moreover, found a good formula for dealing with the virus, seems to be so irrefutable that one simply brushes aside this one drop of wormwood, which so strangely disturbs the conclusiveness of the whole thing, and continues.

The fact that the impulses of the I's enemy, which also affect materialistic medicine or pharmacology by creeping

THE CORONAVIRUS PANDEMIC II

through the most diverse doors that have been opened, among others, by the fact that the idea of the Triformation of the social organism has not taken hold is undeniable, and this problem must be recognized and addressed (even if the opportunity for the for the Triformation impulse is missed for the time being). But to brand the attack on the free I exclusively on this level and to rush past an essential field of attack by this counter-spirit with flags flying because of ignorance of the super-sensory facts, does not lead only to being dangerously sure of one's cause and thus falling into the knowledge trap after all, but it also leads to the fact that one puts others unnecessarily in danger by careless behavior (which one is sure is not careless, because of the irrefutable conviction that others cannot be endangered by a "harmless" virus). If the actual origin of the virus (spiritually sleeping humanity!) as well as the manipulator of this particle ("Soratic" counter-spirituality) remain unknown, one may start with "right" but arrive sometimes at "wrong." One insists on the correctness of the equation, but doesn't notice that the "signs" in the equation have suddenly changed.

For this reason, one of the biggest problems we have today concerning the Sars-CoV-2 virus is once again emphasized:

Yes, it is the *human being* who grants the virus entrance as part of his life. And the physical body evades – under the guidance of the "sleeping" I, that is, the higher I that has not become conscious in the physical body – the Sars-CoV-2 virus, as it has always done in the past, when the human organism came into contact with other pathogens. This means that the human being takes a pathogen with the Sars-Cov-2-Virus into his organism in the customary way – namely unconsciously – which, however, cannot be treated in the customary way by a "sleeping" I, something recognizable by the immune system's strong reaction, which can lead to the most severe effects of the disease. The virus manages to take the "peripheral" I (if one wishes to use to the terminology of some authors) by surprise, which the human being, due to his spiritual neglect, has not brought into his inner being and made conscious there, letting it stay asleep, so to speak, and provoking it to a kind of autoimmune reaction.

The unconscious or subconscious contact with *this* pathogen is no longer sufficient. What man has neglected in his spiritual development, namely the conscious striving for access to his higher I, now comes back at him as a spiritual fact with manifold potency in the form of a particle (corresponding to his materialistic thinking and his conviction that the world is a particle-cosmos). And he can only overcome this if he (contrary to the materialistic particle-cosmos conviction) establishes a fully conscious access to his higher I and thus elevates the imperishable I to the fully responsible, powerful controller of his self as well as that of all immunological processes in his bodily organism.

That man with the best will is not able to do this, belongs to the great misery which humanity has prepared for itself and from which it can no longer emerge unscathed. (This is the price of total freedom of the human I: that real consequences result from man's actions, from which he will not be redeemed by a deus ex machina. For he must realize that he himself is the deus ex machina. He is the free divine being in whom the good spiritual world places its trust. No higher power will come to sweep up the heap of shards he has produced. The Redeemer was already here! Man must recognize and learn to use the tools assigned to him through the Redeemer's sacrifice.)

Therefore, what we integrate into our organism, in this case with Sars-CoV-2, is treated by our organism at first in the same way as before, but since it differs from before in its spirit (by the fact that humanity has let it become a real effective danger by the will to be spiritless, and it being moreover the carrier of the Sorat impulse), no "automatic" protection is provided now against such pathogens, as it was potentially before – depending on what lay in the karma of the individual. What has now become a part of human life in the form of the coronavirus has – at least when seen from a good-divine view – has not been conceived of as such a part, and it has not suffered, as in former times, the products of Lucifer or Ahriman as a somewhat unpleasant "aid" to the awakening of knowledge from a higher point of view. It is now a particle – as bearer of the "counter-I-spirituality" – that has become a part of human life, which as emanation and expression of human free will rejects the living spirit-mechanism in the physical organism, making it unable to act or, expressed differently, which no longer allows the spirit-mechanism to interact with that particle, or more exactly the "spirit" of that particle, in an adequate, "natural," beneficial way for humanity. The equation is the same. But, as said before, the constants of its terms carry reversed signs – which in the real world can mean the result is upside-down.

What we have sent out as materialistic thoughts returns now in finer substantiality. It is we ourselves who, after all, live in the region to where we send our thoughts. In this region emerge physical-material manifestations of humanity's materialistic thoughts as metamorphosed products within the present state and form of the world, (which is called the "physical mineral kingdom" in the occult school). So you see how powerful man is now – when applied to the good, In the sense of "the True, the Beautiful and the Good."

For the first time, through the I's freedom, the human being has the ability to work with the physical products of his own spirit. Something has come into being that is really of human creative origin. And man must now deal with this product. (That the primary host of the Sars-CoV-2 virus may have been a bat or some other animal is irrelevant in this respect.) For the first time man has exhausted the potency, which has been given to him as an I-being, to create such a thing. Not in a laboratory! (That can also happen.) A spiritual creation is meant; the creation of a physical product by his psychical-spiritual behavior.

The world is a moral world! All natural phenomena are moral outpourings of spiritual beings.

That is the world. And since man has arrived at the consciousness-soul age he has become, by what the Christ event has given him, responsible for the being and the future of his world. He has responsibility because the ability to bear responsibility has now been given to him. He has borne responsibility for his world since he has been capable of undertaking it. He has become able to decisively shape his world through his I. But the I alone does not guarantee a good development of himself and his world! Through his I he can bring the world to good as well as to bad. He has just as much the power to devastate his world as to lead it to a cosmos of selflessness and creative life. With his fourth component of being (along with his physical body, life-body and soul-body), with his I, this potency has indeed come to shape his world. But something else must now be added to the I and its potency if he would transform his world into a cosmos of selflessness, love, eternal live: *higher morality.*

At this point in our development, the individual human being is given the task of gradually bringing his I *within* his incarnation to just such a consciousness as when he leads his life between death and a new birth. Only then can he come to that "higher morality." This higher morality can only exist through the consciously sought connection to the divine spirit. If the connection remains subconscious (for in reality it is always there), what is carried out on earth by the I may not be "good" either.

If this connection is not actually sought consciously, if one does not acquire through appropriate exercises the means which are needed to clearly recognize what is really "moral" in the sense of the divine spirit, who wants to see us grow to be his equal for our own good, then the higher I remains unconsciously active in the incarnation. In the end, however, the actual greatness and mission of the I is, as it were, extinguished. In that case, the human being could just as well have remained a being without the I. He would then have only a physical body, an etheric-body and an astral-body, and he could advance at most to intellectual- or-sensitivity-soul in his development. But there is a serious difference between the times before the Christ-event and before the consciousness-soul age: *Previously he didn't have such an I at his disposal* with which he could entirely control his lower components-of-being. But now he has it. And that means: If he treats himself and the world as if he didn't have this I he is guilty toward his own spirit and the spirit of the world. Now he commits spiritual failings and wrongdoings, no longer "only" psychical ones.

And at this point is where the spiritual being can gain access who not only mostly rages in the astral-body like the Luciferic spirits or like the Ahrimanic spirits mostly in the etheric-body, but the one that can be called the *I-enemy*.

The door and gate are opened to it by the spiritual failings of man, by the failures of the I. And in the case of the coronavirus this happens in that the spiritual failures of the human-I, which in this phase of the world context has fallen though continual repetition into materialization, not only in the thought-ether, but has also left its mark on the physical plane, condensed so to speak, to be used as the bearer for slipping into the component-members-organism of man – in the dress of Asuric substantiality. Matter is prepared in an amoral way by the Asuras to be the bearer of Soratic impulses against the I. Man is totally unconscious of this attack against his spiritual nature. His organism reacts as it usually does. But it is now dealing with a substantiality that it cannot cope with in the usual way. If this fact is not recognized, it will also not be understood that this virus is so terrible not primarily because it leads to certain diseases of the physical body or even to death, but because it is a gateway for the impulses of the counter-I-entity in the spiritual part of man; because then man is threatened to substitute his spiritual part for material earthly existence. It would be counteracting the deed of Christ. But that would mean: the falling of man *below* the lowest point of his natural descent from spiritual heights to the physical/material plane. Something begins (unforeseen in the good-divine world-plan) which can be described as damaging the actual human being's core, the I. (Rudolf Steiner mentioned this phenomenon in "Geisteswissenschaftlichen Menschenkunde," GA 107, pg. 266). And with this dreadful counter-development, which is the will of the Counter-I-entity, a first victory has been won by the Sars-CoV virus as the "Advance guard" of this entity's army.

The Consequences of a Covid-19 Infection

When speaking of the "inability to act" of the spirit--
mechanisms of the higher I, or of no longer being able to act
adequately, this means that every adult person infected with
the Sars-CoV-2 virus in whom the I – around 21 years of age
– can fully enter into its function in the human organism, will
have to deal in one way or another with the effects of meeting
with that "counter-spirituality" particle, whether noticed or
not (And I may add that if it is not noticed, it would in most
cases not be an advantage from a spiritual point of view).

Due to the measures that have been taken to avert the
spread of infection on a larger scale, there are dramatic
consequences for countless people, the effects of which are
not yet foreseeable. Starting with mental disturbances, which
run through all age groups, but which probably affect
children and the elderly the most. The economic
consequences are obvious; how societies as such develop in
their respective internal organisms, that is, how people react
among themselves and toward each other, is put to the test;
and that national-chauvinistic or "economic- chauvinistic"
tendencies are emerging in countries and peoples can

already be seen in the distribution of vaccines – whatever one may personally think of vaccination itself – (the vaccines that are sent, if at all, by the economically prosperous countries to the poorer countries are those which their own populations do not prefer.) And surely there are many other consequences that have resulted from the rules and precautions taken to contain the pandemic that will be seen and felt in the future.

In addition to these catastrophes, another one is now looming which is directly related to the virus: Aside from the suffering of those who have experienced a disruption in their lives due to the illness caused by Covid-19, apart from those people who lost their lives due to the Covid-19 disease, which – as indicated in the first volume – might represent "interference" with individual karma, and apart from those who also suffer through the loss of a loved one, the physical, psychological and spiritual *long-term* consequences of a Sars-CoV-2 infection will assume tremendous significance.

It is not possible to thoroughly address the consequences of such an encounter of this counter-spirituality with the I of an unprepared person within the framework of this short book, which can only illuminate a few aspects, and barely touch upon them.

The fact that a growing proportion of formerly infected persons – regardless of whether the course of the initial disease was severe, mild, or asymptomatic – are affected by a so-called *long covid* or *post covid* syndrome, indicates the lasting effects caused by the infection, (which, incidentally, do not happen in influenza virus infections, with which the Sars-CoV-2 infection is often compared or equated. An Influenza infection can also be severe and even fatal, but once the disease is over the symptoms do not persist and serious damage and impairments of various kinds do *not* occur at a much later point in time as a result of the original disease).

It is self-evident in an epoch of development of humanity, in which the single human soul is to find the entry-point to its higher development through *thinking*, that is, over the bridge of *understanding*, of *insight* into the communications of super-sensory facts, that it is just this entry-point that can be severely handicapped by an injury to the thinking organ or by damage to the nerves, which can occur as a consequence of the Covid-19 disease. The damage thus extends from the respiratory problems of acute illness (cf. Volume I) in a later stage, when the acute illness is believed to have ended, to those areas from which – considered from the viewpoint of humanity as a whole – the initial "sinning" originated. It can result in difficulties concentrating, weakness in remembering, word-finding disorders, and even to declining intelligence, that is, dementia-like symptoms.

But spiritually considered, these symptoms are caused by the I being under attack. This I is destined to take over the leadership of the lower component-members. In the present stage of the development of humanity it has first of all the task of taking over the fully conscious guidance of the astral body, i.e. of the soul. When this is one day fully accomplished, this guidance of consciousness will gradually extend to the etheric body. And when man ascends to his highest level of existence, his I also gains full power of consciousness over his physical body. Since an attack takes place on the I by what one could also call the "anti-I-spirit," which has sought the Sars-CoV-2 virus as a suitable carrier medium, the cause for the consequential damages of the infection occurring in the nerve-sense-system of the human being is to be sought here, namely in the I under attack. But since the I is the highest component-member of the human being and – whether from "without" or "within," unconsciously or consciously for the incarnated human being – the administrator and shape-giver of all the component-members, ultimately all the component members (and thus also all members of the physical body), it can be affected by injury.

There has already been talk of an autoimmune reaction. Due to this unequal altercation with the spirituality of the Sars-CoV-2-virus, a weakening of the I takes place, not only in relation to its guidance of the lower component-members, but also in its actual function toward the organism. The I is attacked and manipulated in such a way that it doesn't protect and ennoble its lower component-members, but assaults and demolishes them. The I, spoken simply, is brought by the I-opponent to do the opposite of what its actual nature and task is. Since the I does not only stand above the *physical* body, but also above the etheric and astral bodies, it has a damaging effect on these component-members when it is brought to act in this opposing way. Thus, the human being does not "only" develop a multi-organ illness which, depending on individual conditions, affects the most diverse areas of the physical body, but he also potentially has to struggle with the effects on his astral and etheric bodies. This can lead to feelings of being overwhelmed, depression, anxiety and personality changes, as well as the feeling of no longer being who one actually is. These phenomena can also come at a later point of time in life, or they can ebb and flow insidiously. And also the uncertainty of not knowing what the course of the illness will be means a successive attrition of the soul.

Now comes the vehemence which can be connected to an attack on the I and which must be borne. If one doesn't recognize this spiritual dimension and – as is currently widespread within the anthroposophical movement – thinks that a Covid-19 infection consists of more or less serious "common cold symptoms," then one is looking (with a most limited view) only at the physical symptoms that appear during the acute phase of the illness. Because he knows about reincarnation, the anthroposophist could be inclined to say to himself: *I don't care as much about the physical body as the materialist does. For me spiritual development is important! So it's not so important to me if the physical body in this life is damaged or not. I'll be getting a new one in the next life anyway.* This would be a doubly short-sighted viewpoint!

This attitude may have a certain justification, but of course the anthroposophical spiritual student in particular will strive to take adequate care of his physical body as well, because he knows that the human being can only fulfill his life tasks, which he has undertaken in the spiritual world during prenatal existence, if he does not negligently ruin his physical body. The human being needs the physical body to fulfill his karmic tasks. And the other part of the doubly short-sighted view consists of not realizing that in this case he is involved with something that exceeds the challenge to his physical body. The damage goes far beyond the purely physical damage that can be observed. Here for the first time in the development of humanity, the I is directly threatened in this specific way in its actual, higher function. It is about damage to the higher forces of consciousness!

If the I cannot readily, or can no longer fully assume its actual function, it is much more difficult for the person concerned to follow the training path of spiritual self-education, or to be open to the spiritual worlds at all. Achieving higher consciousness development will become even harder for the human being compared to the conditions already made difficult by materialistic thinking. And for those who have already achieved it, meditation will certainly not be easier at first. They will have to struggle greatly so that the I becomes master over the lower soul-components, because it is really an attack on the I, even if it takes place via the domain of the asuras, via the gateway of the physical body, via damage to the physical body. When the I is attacked, it affects all the other component members. So just as the I is able to become master of the lower component-members in the best sense, if it is weak powerful effects on the lower component-members also emanate from it. For this weakness affects the other component-members of man with just as much negative, destructive strength as his moral maturity can have the strongest positive effects on the other component members. If the master in the house gets weak and sick, everything becomes disorderly.

The I enables the human being to live selflessly. *Selflessness* is a gift to the human environment, it is the water of life for the whole human organism. For this the I has been given to humanity. Selflessness is the actual quality of the I, to which it is destined. But it can only be received or unfolded by means of the human being's free decision. But because neglect has occurred in the I's development, the scourge known as Covid-19 is a phenomenon that affects the whole of humanity. What good could be brought forth for the human organism through the selflessness of the I, is reversed by the neglect of the I and now has an effect on the human organism in a bad sense, that is, as a "pandemic." (This neglect was, so to speak, the origin of the virus.) Therefore, it is also a phenomenon that crisscrosses individual karma (see volume 1, page 24ff). And for the same reason, one should not commit the error of thinking that the people who become ill from Covid-19 are not strong in their I for karmic reasons. It may very well happen that people who have not yet begun consciousness-soul activity fall ill with Covid-19. But this neglect is a "humanity-epochal" neglect, which is why also those souls who have begun to achieve a consciousness-soul awakening in any way (not necessarily the anthroposophical path of training), are likewise not protected from the disease of Covid-19 and its consequences. As it is characteristic for "humanity-epochal" neglect, those who have contributed least to this neglect are also affected. Such souls then share – as somewhat innocent, but not necessarily voluntary victims – in their individual karma the consequences of the karma of humanity. If one wishes to understand the spiritual dimension of the Coronavirus problem, one must also keep in mind that – as already mentioned above and emphasized once more here – that when dealing with neglect involving the I, humanity risks having the rug being pulled out from under the effectiveness of its own spiritual inspiration, sent to it from the spiritual world, because the physical conditions for its effectiveness are made more difficult or are withdrawn.

The Psychical-Spiritual Path of Schooling and Its Effects

Man has been freed to freedom, and this has a price. It can lead to uncomfortable consequences if one doesn't want to "go to school," but thinks that he is already mature enough with what he has. A critical point in human evolution has been reached. A great chance exists for us, which, if we use it, will determine the whole course of the world's development and can lead us, together with the created world, back to unification with the Logos at the end of our own development. The chance exists today to take the first steps toward "deification," through the I becoming conscious in the physical body, that is, during the incarnation, and it is precisely for this reason that at the same time the frontal attack on this chance is undertaken against the I becoming conscious, by spirits that do not want to enter into union with the Logos, but instead to realize their selfhood in eternity at the expense of the forces of other beings, such as those of humanity. They try to manipulate man in such a way that he does not realize that he is excluded – that in the end he only serves for the realization of alien, inscrutable will impulses – by that "organ" in him being affected with which he would be able to notice this and prevent it: his I, his component which is in the actual sense godlike. It is an attempt to make God's creatures ungodly and torpedo the possibility of those creatures becoming creators (in the sense of their Creator, the divine spirit of selflessness, love, truth and life).

The fact that on the one hand the great chance exists for man, through his godlike component, to develop in his total being to a god, and that on the other hand it is just this development that certain elements want to prevent by any means, is something that man must learn to recognize. And above all, he must learn to see it *today* and want to learn to see it if he wants to be an anthroposophical spiritual student. For otherwise he risks that spiritual science itself or, more accurately, fragments of spiritual science, are misunderstood or misused and become through him the destructive instrument that is at the service of that frontal attack on man's chance for higher consciousness. This can happen if anthroposophical spiritual-science is misunderstood at its core. And it is this core which must be apprehended by whoever wants to be a spiritual student of Anthroposophy. In doing so, he would first have to realize, would have to freely and openly admit, that by means of the repeatedly mentioned "method," with which in the anthroposophical movement one so often proceeds today to judge certain events, what is correct may be recognized and repeated, but that the conclusions drawn do not necessarily lead to correct results when earthly logic alone is used. This method may even lead to the opposite of what is revealed to be true in the light of spiritual reality. Here, therefore, caution should be exercised.

For one should, or must, as an anthroposophical spiritual student, reflect on what is *the core of anthroposophical spiritual research*: It is what is called the *training path of the soul*.

If one admits that in reality he does not have the means to super-sensibly investigate the still unknown phenomena in the world, such as the Coronavirus (which is why the above-mentioned "method" is resorted to), one should by no means throw in the towel, for he knows that a remedy is available!

The basis for solving almost all the problems that are currently dominant in humanity is the consistent education of one's own soul. A person is truly an anthroposophist or, expressed differently, an anthroposophical spiritual *student*, only if he engages in the training of the soul for which Rudolf Steiner gave specific details, and doesn't stand still at the beginning but wants to advance, that is, if he learns to identify the mistakes he has made and then to correct them, and if he is willing to learn new things and, if necessary, to say goodbye to old ideas if they turn out to be imperfect; if he also really practices with seriousness, dedication and diligence.

If by his psychical actions (by thinking, feeling and willing impulses) the human being can undertake changes in the world, including physical conditions as is the case now not only with the coronavirus, as a result of his materialistic thinking practiced for decades, he must seek the means to purify these psychical actions and to channel them constructively!

A constructive shaping of the world can succeed by mastering the still largely subconscious soul. And this mastery in turn occurs (gradually and depending on the individual's condition and possibilities) by working through the corresponding soul exercises; by giving these exercises a *central place* in everyday life, and by defending this place against the storms of the everyday sensory world, because one knows that he will only be able to persevere in such storms by not stopping the exercises, but by continuing them steadfastly. There is something very special about these exercises of the soul, about the self-education of one's own soul, which (unlike when the child enters a conventional school) can only come from the conscious will of the mature individual: If one practices to purify one's own soul in its various activities of thinking, feeling and willing, if one practices purposefully and constantly to become a "better person," so to speak, at some point effects occur in a completely different domain than the one in which the exercises were performed and to which the exercises applied, namely the domain of the soul. As a result of the soul's self-education an innovation in the domain of the *spirit* occurs! An awakening of consciousness of the world of higher truth and reality results. By means of the *exercises on the soul* the capacity for super-sensory knowledge, for unimagined spiritual powers develop! (For this reason Rudolf Steiner named his exercise guide for psychical self-education: *"Knowledge of Higher worlds and its Attainment."*

The ability that one would like to possess in order to to make serious statements about the nature of the coronavirus and the phenomenon's related effects and developments, the ability which would replace the questionable method of "logically" compiling the results of research by third parties which do not refer to the present situation and throwing them together with statistical surveys and all kinds of other assertions not drawn from anthroposophical spiritual knowledge into a questionable potpourri, that ability is to be acquired by the serious, devoted and constant performance of modest-seeming soul exercises. Certainly the more spiritual the view which is able to illuminate knowledge of the phenomena, the more conscientiously and courageously must be practiced. This also means that one must not let oneself be upset by failure and that one must above all be ready to sincerely face oneself again and again.

Unfortunately these two conditions are often not fulfilled, which results in one "realizing" that the path of practicing self-education of the soul is correct and necessary, but prefers to walk the path in theory, which in reality means not at all. For yes: one cannot avoid having quite unpleasant experiences on this path of practice with the depth of one's own soul and sometimes also arriving at disappointing insights about one's own nature – insights which, however, only disappoint the ego, which is extremely salutary and the most important step towards the acquisition of spirit-knowledge. The anthroposophist knows that this path exists and that it truly leads to new and marvelous qualities of consciousness and abilities (among other things). And because he knows about it and therefore can also see what possibilities are opened to humanity by the fact that individuals begin to open sources from which great benefits can flow for many, he is, in a way, obliged to use this path. It is of course in a person's karma if he or she feels attracted to Anthroposophy. It is no coincidence if his destiny leads him to be fascinated by spiritual-scientific knowledge of the world and humanity. His higher I has set the track in prenatal existence for him to enjoy the privilege in earthly life of becoming acquainted now with fundamental truths that may come to humanity more extensively in the future. But this does not come to him purely for pleasure. To become acquainted with super- sensory knowledge is not the same as with earthly knowledge. This "privilege" of destiny comes to a person only because of his great interest in the super-sensory insights which have been achieved by another before him, and have now become clear to him, which tap with their truth into the truth in his own interior and open up perspectives for him (which for others have not yet opened) to use his own will to walk the training path of the soul, which leads to the ability to independently recognize spiritual realities, and never to deviate from it, even if this sometimes means deprivation and suffering for the lower self. For a person whose path of destiny has led him to anthroposophy, this path of practice must be by far the most important compared to other anthroposophical activities. For he knows that in this way he can "prove" himself to the divine-spiritual world which speaks to him through anthroposophical messages and which he admires and reveres with all his soul for the trust it has placed in him. The path of practice is also the means to prove himself a useful helper of the good, the good spirit, and to be equipped for such a contribution. He knows that in reality he can only serve the development of the world as a whole by the ennoblement of his soul.

And it is because such a person knows this fact that he understands Christ's words are meant for him: *"From everyone to whom much has been given, much will be required; and from the one to whom much has been entrusted, even more will be demanded."* (Luke 12,48)

If, therefore, the present disaster is caused by the burdening of the general thoughts-ether with untrue thoughts, namely with thoughts of a purely material world, then it is the task of humanity, but above all of that individual who rightly wants to call himself an anthroposophist, to suffuse this thoughts-ether with *true* thoughts.

What are these true thoughts?

They are the thoughts about the origin and context of the world with that being who is called the *Logos* in the prologue to the Gospel of John; the thoughts about that Logos, the creator *"Word,"* from whom everything came forth and who became the *"life,"* then the *"Light"* for humanity, before He finally became *"Flesh,"* in order to remove the sting of death by His sacrifice – passing through fleshly, material death – thus giving man the ability to reach full consciousness of the factual immortality of his spiritual being. And, from this consciousness, to rise out of free will to complete immortality, to the immortality of his whole being by the interspersion of his component-members with the moral principles of the Logos. These principles, which have been revealed to humanity through the life and deeds of the Logos on earth in the form of the Christ Jesus, are: impartiality (the strength of devotion to the eternal and the good in the individual), love and conscience. If these true thoughts stir in his soul, the person is drawn to the principles of the Logos. He purifies his soul through the application of the moral principles of the Logos, for which he has many opportunities in everyday life. It becomes light in him. The "moralizing" of his thoughts, however, is also the beginning of the moralization of the general thoughts- ether, in which all human beings are related to each other.

The human being treading the path of soul-exercise "revives" this thoughts-ether, which today must seem almost dead to super-sensory consciousness. In this way he lets a healing serum flow into the world, from which *all* people benefit. Through this, however, nothing less happens than that man takes the same path – only in reverse – that the Logos once took to him. The human being rises from his mere "carnal being" to the "*light*," which is the enlightenment of his consciousness, the enlivening of the thought-ether by those very exercises, by practicing to think true thoughts of the Logos, of the Christ. Thereby the "Light" itself, the "Holy Spirit" comes to him.

He becomes a light-source through this Light, which is kindled in his individual inner self and which radiates out into the world, through which he illuminates the general thought-ether with the light of truth. It is the only permanently effective means against the various spawns of "evil," the only possibility above all to prevent the mass appearance of *new* spawns of this counter-spirit impulse.

For this reason, because the person who has come to Anthroposophy knows about these contexts, because he knows how he can take precautions against such manifestations of evil in the world and how he can instead lead himself and his world to moral ennoblement, to truth and to life, makes such a person ultimately guiltier if he does not seize the means known to him for the preservation and evolution of the world with all seriousness, than a person who adheres to the materialistic worldview and behaves accordingly, but who has never heard anything about all this. The anthroposophical spiritual student, the disciple of Christ, must tell himself again and again that he is not yet of service to the world through the knowledge of certain elements alone. Only when these elements of knowledge are impressed on his soul in such a way that he becomes an "other" person in whom these elements of truth are awoken to life, namely by unsparing honesty toward the "shallowness" of his own soul and the relentless effort to rectify it, will he do justice to the gift of his incarnation and his karmic mission. Not by knowing alone, but by the

THE CORONAVIRUS PANDEMIC II

transformation of his inner self to the good. The counter-spiritual forces also impart knowledge! (Although it then becomes a weapon against the person himself.)

How consistently one can and should go on this path and what means he can use is made clear by the parable of Jesus Christ "about the unjust steward" in the Gospel of Luke. (A short interpretation of this parable is included in the appendix.)

The person who seeks the path to betterment of the world reaches real knowledge, that is knowledge of the causes and contexts of the circumstances and phenomena surrounding him, through exercises of the soul that are based on the moral principles of the Logos-Christ. In this way he can also gain real insight into the "nature" of the coronavirus and the complexity and challenges created by it, without having to settle for mere belief and clever combinations of circumstantial evidence.

One will then realize that to believe in love and in the immeasurable healing powers in the human being alone, to which people like to refer today (also within the anthroposophical movement), nothing is done, and that the belief in the free, autonomous human being does mean doing or not doing within the social context, the social organism, whatever makes sense to you at the moment, but that it's rather a matter of *"love of inner freedom,"* that is, freedom from one's own particular point of view. (GA 10, 25) Then one will be in a position to discover the *actual* danger posed by this virus.

For the spiritual-scientist, infection with the coronavirus means a serious danger for humanity at this point in its psychical-spiritual development. When we look at the nexus of the pandemic emergence with spiritual insight, we clearly recognize that what the human being takes in with the Sars-CoV-2 virus itself is *not* something which he *should* take in, because it actually should not be there and for this reason he cannot favorably process it in the usual way that has been possible until recently. The spiritual scientist considers an infection with the coronavirus dangerous for a different reason than does the conventional natural scientist (Although he also cannot overlook the suffering of those fallen ill and the tragic, interrupted karmic destiny of the dead who the virus has claimed and will continue to claim. He cannot accept this tragic development with the attitude that is displayed by so many contemporaries today, that beyond the – doubtless justified – pointing to the psychological, social and economic consequences of the political measures taken to contain the pandemic, the fate of the sick and the dead fades into the background with the erroneous and, moreover, downright cynical argument that there are much worse diseases or events in the world and that it is, after all, the karma of the individual if he falls ill or dies. If the sick and the dead are not enough for some to speak of a "pandemic," then let them bear in mind that the Being who has usurped the coronavirus phenomenon has intelligence par excellence, and that everything, really everything, is considered and finely worked out by that entity. This includes, of course, the fact that the Sars-Cov-2 virus, compared to what was already there and even more so to what is yet to come, outwardly appears "harmless." It is the vanguard of something quite different. But it already carries the same spiritual signature).

Whoever is able to see all this, however, cannot avoid recognizing that humanity has reached the limits of its possibilities by the appearance of such a counter-spiritual bearer as the Sars-Cov-2-virus. For if it is only possible to acquire the means to fortify oneself against such attacks through spiritual maturity, that is, through consistent and untiring treading the path of spiritual training, then one must realize that he has not yet developed these means at all, and that in addition to the will to develop them, one needs above all one other thing to be able to do so: *Time.*

A characteristic phenomenon of these times is an activity of the so-called Ahrimanic spirits – aphoristically spoken: the distortion of time, namely the acceleration of the development processes of all physical-sensory (or "sub-sensory") things and events. Here the hierarchy of the

Ahrimanic spirits is preparing the groundwork for the counter-I impulse. Because time is running out for us in every conceivable way, for the conditions in which spiritual-soul education must take place are becoming more and more precarious. And now this development is also at risk by the primary physical and soul-spiritual attack referred to here. The karmic path of life can be shortened, so to speak, by the Covid-19 infection.

So what can you do to give yourself the time necessary to bring your spiritual development to where it must be in order to acquire the spiritual instruments for super-sensory knowledge, with which you can be taught about the reality of present and future events and through which you can also acquire the tools to successfully meet the challenges of the present and next cultural epoch without serious harm to spirit, soul and body? What can one do to gain the strength during the present turmoil, which not only strongly challenges the soul, but severely impedes the soul's progress on the moral path of purification leading to spirit-realization, to develop the instruments needed to resist such attacks leading to impairment of the spiritual and psychical organism or the physical body as a result of a Covid-19 infection?

The Black Lodges and the Soul's Training

Unfortunately, in order to approach this topic, you must first make your way through a theme which is a veritable minefield: One must speak (even if here to the least extent possible) of those circles which are consciously at the service of the impulses of the opposing spiritual powers – the circles which Rudolf Steiner (for instance in GA 178) referred to as the "*Lodges of the left hand*" or as "*Occult Brotherhoods,*" which here, in contrast to the "White Lodge" often mentioned by him, will be called "Black Lodges" by me. – Whatever you call them, they exist. Also when today a large part of humanity dismisses this fact as the mother of all conspiracy theories.

But the results of my spiritual research paint a somewhat *different* picture than is drawn by so many people today, who have no doubts about the existence and deplorable willpower of the Black Lodges and who – also within the anthroposophical movement – are active with publications or other comments or appeals, and shape the opinions of a much larger, less "voluble" circle of people.

One of the most important facts to bear in mind with regard to this subject is that today the tendency towards two different paths of development is already beginning to emerge: one path of development that leads to a higher development of man in the sense of the Logos, and another that leads to a descending development. It is most important to note, however, that these two different paths are not represented by the two major "camps" that are so divided today in dealing with the coronavirus. It is not the case, for example, that those who agree today to comply with certain regulations to contain the pandemic are all walking or will walk the downward path, while those who refuse or reject those regulations are on the steep upward path (and vice-versa). It may be that the first group, which trusts conventional natural science and medicine more than the second, is more likely to adhere to the materialistic view of the world and man and ultimately to be misguided by it in making fundamental decisions. However, one must reject the possibility that the group which is skeptical or critical with regard to the statements and guidelines of scientific research, conventional medicine and to a large extent a "predatory capitalistic" economy, will take the path to the higher development, since such an attitude does not necessarily mean that they are striving for *spiritual development* or have a spiritual world and human view at all.

If we stand back a little and look at these things objectively, we might be surprised at first to conclude that there are hardly any fewer people in the second group who lean toward materialism than in the first. For enthusiasm for the protection of the earth and humanity should not be limited to producing less garbage, demonstrating for climate neutrality or consuming only organic food.

Materialism within the second group appears ultimately to be only clothed in a different garment than in the first. Not only in the first group do we find many people who are hoping for a "miracle cure" for the prevention or treatment of covid-19. There are also many who belong to the second group who hope for such a miracle cure, except in the first group they hope to receive it from the hands of conventional science, whereas those in the second group rather expect it to come from alternative medicine or medicinal herbs or even from one of the many kinds of "magic" rituals.

(It is not my intention to only describe my personal opinion here. It does seem to me appropriate, however, to ask that what I say not be interpreted as wanting to applaud conventional natural science and at the same time discredit the impulses that are in the alternative movements, including in the anthroposophical one. Nothing is further from my mind. On the contrary. *If* this book is written for a *personal* reason, it is perhaps to contribute at least a little to the anthroposophical movement's breaking away from any tendency toward sectarianism, radicalism and irrationality, which it has conspicuously succumbed to in the storms of recent times. Strengthening the anthroposophical impulse today means not only living in accordance with Anthroposophy, but also standing up to the aberrations within the anthroposophical movement, and naming them in order to bid them adieu. A weakening of the anthroposophical impulse means to tolerate irrationality and non-spiritual scientific knowledge, as well as sectarian and extremist tendencies. It is precisely my unconditional devotion to the anthroposophical impulse that prompts me to address what is revealed through super-sensory observation of current conditions to be unfavorable to the anthroposophical impulse. I am not at all interested in the protection and prosperity of the materialistic worldview – about which there are already countless critiques in realization to the coronavirus problem – but to that of the *spiritual* worldview. Therefore, this essay mainly deals with the challenges to those human beings who see themselves as anthroposophists or want to become anthroposophists, who, therefore, wish to help the spiritual worldview to triumph in the world. For there are also numerous pitfalls and sink-holes on this path! The spiritual worldview can only be successfully disseminated if one tries to avoid these pitfalls and sink-holes as much as possible).

There are, then, in the second group – in which at present large parts of anthroposophical circles are included – definitely many souls who are also moved by materialistic ideas. In fact, we find here an attitude which, compared to the conventional materialistic attitude, has a particularly unpleasant, namely arrogant note. The search for an alternative means of preventing or curing covid-19 is frequently based on an even more smug, even more presumptuous materialism. The demand not only to be provided with a means that relieves one of the necessity of acquiring the means to deal successfully with the virus and its consequences through psychological and spiritual efforts, but also that this remedy be "pure" of all undesirable effects that one expects from a preparation made by the conventional pharmaceutical industry, is the height of materialism and egoism and is equivalent to the attitude of consuming only organic or Demeter products on principle and under all circumstances, while millions of people in the world – far away – are dying of hunger.

Seeking an alternative remedy is justified and necessary! But from a super-sensible standpoint it should only be done once one has prepared oneself spiritually for the actual reason for Covid-19. And this miracle remedy can really not exist previously. For the real cause of Covid-19 is not physical, and not necessarily psychical, but a *spiritual* problem. Spiritual neglect. This spiritual problem can be solved only by the I, which begins to purify its lower component-members in the course of the aforementioned psychical self-education, which leads to super-sensory knowledge and new abilities. – To work on the *soul* and *spirit* should be the motto of "self-betterment"!

If in recent decades we had only done half as much for the *soul* and *spirit* as for the body, we would have come a long way and would have been able to avert many things that cannot be easily remedied now. Insight into spiritual individual responsibility for the current dilemma must come first. Afterward in some circumstances one may find a remedy which can offer sustainable effective support. Only then, through self-knowledge, will people's eyes be opened for appropriate remedies. – If man should find a cure *before* that, he would be escaping the *test of knowledge*, which alone can initiate a turning point. Therefore, in the final analysis, *every* so-called "remedy" (as well as vaccinations) would not be a gift of the good divine spirit if this insight had not occurred beforehand, or at least in parallel.

Therefore, a person who belongs to the second group is not necessarily a representative of that path of development which in the future leads upwards, toward the Logos. Critical behavior toward the regulations to fight the pandemic does not necessarily and a priori identify someone as a representative of this upward path, which is a spiritual path oriented toward the acquisition of spiritual consciousness. Conversely, one could very well mistakenly assume that the person who has achieved knowledge of the true nature of the Sars-CoV-2-virus through super- sensory insight and is willing to obey certain regulations – which of course today do not derive from super-sensory but from "sensory" considerations – is a representative of the first group. But unlike a representative of the first group and also unlike a representative of the second, he knows that an encounter with the spirituality of this virus would lead to considerable difficulties in his etheric and astral bodies organism, and he would want to spare not only himself but also the people in his surroundings from this destiny. For this reason, as long as there are no other possibilities resulting from psychical-spiritual progress, he would not shrink from the temporary use of a protective mask, for example. For he would recognize the attack on human freedom as being primarily in a completely different domain.

So the two camps of opinion created by the emergence of the coronavirus are not the two developmental paths meant here. Which of these two paths the individual takes depends solely on whether he seeks the Spirit, the living, creative, consciousness-embodying Holy Spirit in the world and in himself, or not. This is all that matters in the choice of paths.

And here one must clearly see that the path of development that winds upward is still a decidedly narrow one. Man has not yet given it much solid ground. Yes, it seems barely built today, almost about to disappear, because the side which was meant to level and stabilize it, so that it could be recognized and entered by a larger number of souls as the right alternative to the huge road that leads in the opposite direction, lacks the commitment that is urgently needed. And the anthroposophical movement belongs to this side. We must always come back to the same, all-important point, on which not only the future of the coronavirus problem hinges, but which is also crucial with regard to countless other factors, by which the earth and its human inhabitants are already acutely threatened. It is the point which, as the foundation of all other activities, should be at the center of the life of a person who wants to be an anthroposophist: It is the *spiritual development*, which, if it wants to be attained on a "white" way, is to be had only through the serious implementation of what the soul encounters on the "path of knowledge" as *soul exercises*.

And it is unfortunately becoming bitterly clear today that a distressingly large portion of the people who count themselves as belonging to the anthroposophical movement obviously do not practice these exercises or do not do so seriously enough. For if they were taken seriously and nurtured everywhere in the anthroposophical movement, one could not get lost in the skirmishes which go on, garnished with all kinds of axioms and facets diametrically opposed to the principles of Christ. We get lost in heated debates, in word-wars about "the truth." We use quotes by Rudolf Steiner, not only to support our own view, but we are actually stealing by using them as a kind of weapon with which to attack the "enemies" of our own opinion, as well winning over the insecure or undecided with the help of this moral dishonesty.

In all this one does not notice that step by step one is in danger of falling into the trap of those forces which consciously and purposefully serve the circles of the so-called Black Lodges. The anthroposophical spiritual student must not fall into this trap!

It must not be overlooked that the attack on human freedom and the spiritual development of humanity comes from two sides. It is a double attack, namely an attack by the virus itself and also an attack in the field of dealing with the virus. As has been pointed out above, through lack of spiritual cognition the first of these two attacks is barely seen, and it is only because of this that the second field of attack, which is meant to divide humanity, can give battle.

Yes, this field (dealing with the virus), is meant to divide humanity! It is the plan of the counter-spiritual powers and the circles that serve them! But the field "dealing with the virus" isn't divided into a good and a bad camp. Instead, this field is divided into two camps, both infiltrated by evil intentions, although in different ways. They oppose each other in group-soul manner, instead of opposing the actual aggressors who continue to act undisturbed – which Rudolf Steiner called "The enemies of knowledge of the present" (GA270, Dornach, pg. 33). These present-day enemies of knowledge are: fear (of what speaks through the reality of the Father-divinity in the world – the world as it has become), hate (of what has come to humanity through the Son of God) and doubt (of the Holy Spirit, through whom thinking can raise itself to super-sensible insight).

Only if man does not concentrate energetically and conscientiously enough on self-education of the soul and is distracted from the *actual task* of contemporary humanity – knowledge of the Son of God's gift and its importance for the further development of humanity – will these enemies of knowledge be allowed to instill their poison in humanity's development.

Then, on the one hand, people will not realize that the attempt to counteract the virus through ever more drastic and at some point permanent intrusion in certain democratically certified so-called fundamental rights, is under the influence of a force that wants to lead humanity into a state of immaturity. And then a different group of people will not realize that opposition to this force in a purely external domain can never be successful, because this force is a *spiritual* force and it achieves its goals precisely by preventing people from developing and using their spiritual potential, by keeping them from serving the good and being fully occupied in the external battlefields. – That it is this power which brings this about must be immediately obvious to every anthroposophical student of the spirit, for on these battlefields – whether on the streets or in one's own family circle – there prevail whipped-up waves of emotion, ranging from rapturous hysteria to contempt for one's fellow human beings.

There is no doubt that the I achieves control of soul-life by means of exercises such as control of thoughts and actions, forbearance and tolerance and impartiality and trust, or the soul's equilibrium.

Where have they gone – the anthroposophical spiritual student's ideals, inflamed by the Christ-spirit?

Of course! One must actively work on earthly conditions! And each individual can only do this to the best of their knowledge and conscience. I am certainly not saying here that one should not be engaged in the various areas where poverty rules! It should be pointed out, however, that even with all the activities in the sensory areas concerning the coronavirus problem, you should be aware that the encounter with the Soratic impulse, which acts via the virus itself as well as via its social consequences, cannot be prevented or overcome by external activities – whether it be by circulars, lectures, protest marches or political or social activities. The only way is by descent into the depths (and abysses) of one's own soul, by the courageous confrontation with oneself, by reflection on the actual primal ground of the human being which lies like a seed waiting to be allowed to germinate; reflection on the spirit through which the potential of the human being can be "unbound" – the only really effective means to cope with the spiritual measures of the counter-spirit. It is a means which *every* person can acquire and use! One is active in the external field in a wholesome way when this activity is characterized by respect for the other person, love, compassion, selflessness, conscience. You don't have to be an initiate to use these means when you are active in the everyday life of the senses, and you don't have to be an initiate to recognize that wherever these moral means are not used or are lacking, the activity cannot be in the sense of the good-divine spirit, but rather in the sense of the spirits opposing Him. The way we *deal* with our opinion proves – no matter what that opinion may be – whether we are really students on the path of exercising the soul, whether or not we are following the Christ-principles that are being embedded in us by these soul-exercises. What the so-called Black Lodges achieve, they do so through *spiritual* work, through immoral *spirituality*. They know very well that the spirit is stronger than the soul and the physical organization and all outer activity. That is why they try in different ways to confuse us, and to dissuade us from our spiritual development, depending on our attitude (whether we are easily inspired by the materialistic worldview or whether we turn to the living Spirit and stand up for humanity's higher development of consciousness). The work of the so-called Black Lodges is beyond question. But today there is a danger of them preying on both opposite areas, not only in the obvious area of the materialistic worldview and natural science, but also at the edge of the area, which is, so to speak, opposite to the former. Souls are tilting away today on both sides of the bridge that leads to soul-balance and the composure of knowledge. As mentioned in the preface, an extensive writing of mine will be published in the foreseeable future about the aims and many intermediate aims of the so-called Black Lodges, about what is being prepared in the background by the Black Lodges concerning the effects of the counter-spiritual powers, and in a framework which I believe gives me the possibility to be able to take responsibility before the reader as well as before the spiritual world to some extent, for approaching and deepening this delicate subject. However, I do not consider this book to be a suitable framework for dealing with this topic exhaustively or in detail.

The Plan of the Black Lodges About Vaccinations

I will only mention a few points that I consider to be essential in the present context:

Humanity as such is on a path of development which leads to materialism in the form of technology, including the human organism itself. To this last point, technology and mechanization, "machinization" of human forces, Rudolf Steiner said that one should not handle these things "by fighting against them." This is "*a completely false view. These things will not fail to happen, they will come. It is only a question of whether they will be staged in the course of world history by people who are selflessly familiar with the great goals of the world, and who will shape these things for the well-being of humanity, or whether the scenario is staged by those groups who exploit these things only in an egotistical or in a group-egotistical sense.*" (GA 178, Dornach, p 218f.)

It is therefore not to be denied that humanity is in a phase of development directed towards the technological domination of the world, including even the forces which lie in the spirit, soul and physical body, and will continue to be so *in the next centuries and millennia.* But on this path of development, in the present and in the near future, it will not be so clear where exactly the activities of the "White Lodge" and where the activities of the "Black Lodges" are, whether what is accomplished in the field of natural science is staged by the Black Lodges. For even if natural science at present is still little instilled with spiritual impulses, or even works completely towards materialism, this does not mean that its work is in the service of a Black Lodge. And in the future this will also be true, that is, not automatically and comprehensively (as can be seen from Rudolf Steiner's statement above). It depends upon whether the natural scientific achievements are used in the sense of the good-divine world plan. If they are carried out in the spirit of the beings who organize this good-divine world plan for the benefit of humanity, then such actions in the sensory world (as those indicated above) will also be sacred services ("sacred" not in the sense of traditional rituals, but as visible testimony to the conscious, freely chosen commitment of the individual human being to the living spirit, to the spiritual knowledge of the world and responsibility for the developments taking place in it).

However, since both sides still in the process of gathering their spiritual forces for what Rudolf Steiner described above for the future, much is still in the "draft stage," and one and the other are undulating into each other. The spiritual paths have not yet separated much from each other, for today people are still beginning to consciously and freely walk *spiritual* paths in the true sense. Black and white are not yet clearly separated from each other. Instead, there is a wide palette of shades and tones. For this reason, and because the spiritual means are still scarcely available, it is extremely difficult to point the finger at certain events or circumstances and identify them as clearly "black" or "white" in origin. Everything is still in the initial stage of the development mentioned here. And everywhere the freedom of the individual I runs through the web of existence, which is continuously woven and can reveal a pattern at the next moment, which was not to be reckoned with at all a short time ago. (For this reason and also because of the fact that the virus as a bearer of the always rigid and constant Soratic impulses – as well as everything else related to it – reacts with great flexibility to human behavior, especially to human spiritual activities, the following is not the final result that is applicable at all times and all places.) It is to be noted that those spiritual forces which oppose the world development plan shaped by the good-divine side in favor of humanity, and which the black lodges serve in one way or another (today the "western" black lodges have a certain preponderance over the "eastern" ones), try to prevent realization of the true human essence by which man would be able to escape their influence and their desire to subjugate. But this happens in a much more sophisticated and ingenious way than could be revealed today to large groups of people who hardly know or even want to know anything about the possibilities and methods of development of the human soul and the human spirit, and about the Christ-impulse and the spiritual science penetrated by this Christ-impulse. If the plans of the counter-spiritual forces, or the Black Lodges, were really so easy to see through, namely by people who, in group-soul-like contexts, let themselves be carried away by a more than dubious "we-feeling" and a resulting extremism towards the supposedly "gullible sheep" or the alleged representatives of evil, if the machinations of the Black Lodges could be stopped by picking out pieces of truth from somewhere and building house- of-cards theories from them, which are then spread by means of "social media" with snowball-like speed – or in other words: *viral* (sic!) – then humanity would hardly have anything to fear from the Black Lodges. Unfortunately, that is not the case.

With regard to the coronavirus problem, the same phenomenon is present and the Black Lodges, because of their basic intention to prevent man's knowledge of his true nature, consequently also want to counteract the development of a medicine that is right for human beings. It is their endeavor to gain control over conventional medicine and other natural-scientific research. Also, to gain control not only over the physical processes, but also over the psychical-spiritual forces of man, which are given to him for the potential control of the physical processes or for further development of them.

With this background, it is impossible to avoid speaking about the most sensitive topic of all, which so heats up the tempers in connection with the coronavirus: *vaccination* against Sars-CoV-2, which promises to protect against falling ill with Covid-19.

It can be determined by means of spiritual observation that with the Sars-CoV-2 virus infection the I of the human being would have to encounter this virus from within the physical body, that is, with the full force of consciousness. In order to completely neutralize the Soratic impulse attached to this virus, we would have to be able to control with full powers of consciousness what is now called the immune system (to control and to direct it), just as we are aware in daytime consciousness of the perceptions in the sensory world. What has occurred by the neglect of the I, and due to the fact that this neglect falls temporally in the third impact of the Soratic entity in the development of humanity, could only be reversed or made completely harmless through the control of certain vegetative processes of the physical organism. But at the present point of development of humanity this is not possible. In addition, man has put a gigantic obstacle in the way of spiritual knowledge by his neglect of his I (which has been the cause of the pathogenic effect of the coronavirus). Additionally, humanity has weakened, reduced its chances of reaching higher knowledge and abilities as quickly as possible. Moreover, humanity experiences today the rapid growth of all sensory processes, a time-shrinking so to speak, while its spiritual development does not keep up with this process of acceleration, but rather stagnates, or is lamed. In view of this as well as the fact that the infection with Sars-CoV-2 and its fatal consequences for the physical, mental-psychical and spiritual organism of the human being is a pandemic event, also from the spiritual point of view, that it therefore represents a karmic concern for the whole of humanity, the few who have actually already set out on the path of soul-spiritual development, or have even progressed further along, must now also recognize that their possibility for fulfilling their spiritual task for humanity is threatened. Like any other human being who has to fulfill their karmic task in life, an infection with Sars- CoV-2 would also put a huge obstacle in their way toward fulfilling their karmic task. If the karmic task of those few individuals already extends to not only advancing their *own* development, but also as an "instrument" prepared by the higher spirits to give decisive spiritual help to humanity, could *not* come to humanity, however, and would be bitterly missing if their component members – physical-body, life-body, astral body, I – organization is impaired by the consequences of the infection.

So what can be done?

At this point, it is only possible to speak of something that can only be of value if it is received with the necessary impartiality and peace of mind. It is the intention of the so-called Black Lodges to strive as quickly as possible and ever more "perfectly" for the command over those processes, those forces, which are connected with the birth of man, with the maintenance of his physical organs' activity and with death. Very special attention is paid to the command and specific manipulation of the mysteries of the genetic structure of the physical body, in which the whole karmic plan of humanity is worked into by the prenatal I and by the spiritual hierarchies standing alongside this I; this means the immoral manipulation of the prenatal and postnatal human DNA.

It is the case, however, that what is envisioned has not yet been achieved. It is true that much has already been achieved today towards this development. But it is still far from Rudolf

Steiner's relevant remarks or – clothed in mystery language – in the *Revelation of John.*

This is because the corresponding natural-scientific branches, whose expertise is needed for such undertakings, are by no means fully under the direction of the Black Lodges. It would not only be naive and inaccurate, but also slanderous to accuse natural science per se of being influenced by the Black Lodges. In the future – if mankind does not completely erase spiritual knowledge – more and more of the morally good impulses of a spiritual science will shine on the natural scientific fields of research – even if only selectively or in smaller areas.

The Black Lodges do not yet have science at the point where they want it to be in respect to DNA manipulation in order to impede the "Lord of Karma," Christ, from doing his selfless and loving work on the development of the individual human soul. But they are getting close.

The mRNA vaccination, especially criticized by the anthroposophical side and regarded as a pathogenic or even deadly work of the devil, differs essentially from the earlier, classical vaccinations in that the human organism is not brought into contact with the virus itself or with parts of the virus, but only with the "blueprint" for the distinctive viral envelope, that is, for the so-called surface, in this case the "spike" protein. This is considered to be a major advance by conventional virology because – in contrast to live vaccines – the human organism is not exposed to the onslaught of the actual pathogen.

The principle of immunization itself, which, by the way, does not in principle speak against the anthroposophical view, is based on a careful acquaintance of the human being with the pathogen or with parts of this pathogen. So it can be assumed that by vaccination the human being goes through the natural infection on a small scale, so to speak. He is then already forearmed for a possible encounter with the pathogen. If today some voices from the circle of the anthroposophical movement claim that only a direct infection with a pathogen can be of value for humans, it must be countered from a spiritual- scientific perspective that in the case of the Sars-CoV-2 virus this, however, leads to catastrophe. (What is coherent and justified in itself is now, as said before, turned upside down by a "change of signs.") If one lets it come to an infection with Sars-CoV-2, not what would have been expected earlier happens. The "peripheral" I is deceived, as it were, and at some point begins to fight its own organism – the physical as well as the psychical organism.

Could vaccination against the coronavirus (especially with the mRNA vaccine), which is introduced by an element which does not want to know anything about spiritual knowledge of the virus and also of the human being, which looks at the problem materialistically and not holistically, be "coincidentally" the solution to the problem?

Certainly not!

To be sure, it should not and can in no way be claimed that all those people who were and are involved in the development and deployment of a vaccine against the coronavirus are working on behalf of the Black Lodges. Most of them are undoubtedly animated by the honest desire to help and to bring with their activity something good for humanity, through which a "normal" life can again be possible. (It is needless to mention again here that a "normal" life, as people knew it before, will no longer exist – neither by means of such a vaccination nor some other preparation or "natural" miracle remedy.) But even if today many people in the corresponding research areas have good intentions, it is nevertheless true that the Black Lodges clearly intend to achieve their *actual gambit* by means of the mRNA vaccination against the coronavirus.

Based on extrasensory perception, as well as sensory observations, I conclude that I *cannot confirm* the catastrophically negative effect on the human organism that some anthroposophists, and others, have attributed to this vaccination against Sars-CoV-2.

THE CORONAVIRUS PANDEMIC II

Due to the short time-span of just under one and a half years that have passed since the first clinical studies, it is not yet possible to say conclusively from a natural-scientific point of view whether, and if so, how the vaccination will affect the human organism in the long-term in respect to any undesirable side effects. From the spiritual-scientific side, taking into consideration the possibility of an imperfect or incorrect extrasensory "seeing" of these connections by me, and the events being still in development, it can be stated that in any case such side effects as those that occur as long-term consequences of a Covid-19 illness, namely a physical and psychical-spiritual impairment, or even that a manipulation of the psychical-spiritual organism were intended through this vaccination, *neither* occur unintentionally as an unknown side effect or long-term side effect, *nor* are they *currently intended* by the Black Lodges. – And according to my spiritual observation of the state of affairs, the perfidious plan of the Black Lodge consists of just this! I will describe it here now in few words.

Even though, as previously mentioned, it has only been a fairly short period of time since the first tests of the vaccination, it must already be admitted that a widespread catastrophe in terms of negative after-effects due to the vaccination has failed to materialize. By today's date (8.15.2021), just under two billion people have been fully vaccinated. Almost 4.7 billion vaccine doses have been administered in total. If the vaccination had resulted in the consequences that were feared by the anthroposophical side, it would not have been possible to prevent this from becoming known, no matter how closely the press was controlled. Because by now almost everyone knows someone who has already been vaccinated, and they can see from their own observations that the great catastrophe has not materialized.

As with any other vaccination, there are also with the coronavirus vaccination so-called vaccination harm, serious illnesses that have clearly occurred in people as a result of the vaccination, and these are in no way to be ignored or downplayed here. But compared to many other vaccinations that have been carried out for a long time, such problems occur relatively seldom in the case of the vaccination against the Sars- CoV-2 virus.

Even before the first vaccines were approved, my spiritual research led to what is now generally confirmed, also by my "sensory" observation: that this mRNA vaccination, in which the entire information is not transmitted by the virus which, as a bearer of the Soratic impulse, has the previously described fatal consequences for the human being, but only a copy of the blueprint of the viral envelope (so that the human immune system builds up a defensive phalanx against the garment of the virus in which it wraps itself, preventing an absorption of the entire viral information into the human cell, without the human being having to come into contact with the entire virus beforehand) prevents the main spiritual damage that occurs as a result of an infection, and therefore does not lead to such consequences as were to be feared or are today cited by certain people as having allegedly occurred. In observing many people in my own environment who have been vaccinated twice (approximately 100), they have had no difficulties, if we exclude the initial reaction to the vaccination, which can occur due to the successful activation of the so-called acquired immune system, which can sometimes occur after the second vaccination (such as temporary fever, chills or aching limbs). I could not find any other changes in the human organism (neither physical nor psychical-spiritual), that could lead me to agree with the opinion that spiritual activity is no longer possible after vaccination or only limited due to its terrible side effects.

(I would like to mention, however, that one of the few people I know and whom I trust to make a spiritual assessment of the current situation, namely José Martinez, who, by the way, shares my assessment of the Soratic nature of the Sars-CoV-2 virus, has told me of other observations. He had encountered people who, after vaccination – whether after an initial vaccination or a complete vaccination remained unclear – experienced a wide range of side effects, such as disorientation, equilibrium problems, concentration difficulties or panic attacks – all symptoms that are characteristic of a long-covid or post-covid syndrome. José Martinez, based on his own observations of those so affected, is convinced that the vaccination leads to similar problems as an infection with the virus itself. Because of my great respect for the results of José Martinez's research and success with diverse action in other fields, I did not want to let this report be swept under the table. Nor do I wish to imply that there is an error in his rendering. But when I am asked about this question, I can only state what has been made known to me by extrasensory means, and what has been confirmed by my perceptions in everyday sensory life. Although I am neither a physician nor a natural health professional, people have turned to me again and again in considerable numbers with the most diverse questions about health, or rather illness, with questions about a specific health problem. Until now, however, no one has contacted me who feels that he or she has been lastingly damaged in any way as a result of a vaccination. This complements my own observations in my family and acquaintance circles, also in the anthroposophical one.)

So I can also *not* confirm, both from the spiritual (about which I will speak in a moment) and from the sensory consideration of circumstances, numerous deaths of people as a result of the vaccination.

It could happen, however, that with an early development of the soul-spiritual capacities one has found something that is perhaps basically correct, thus worth communicating, but one is unable to support it by current spiritual-scientific research nor by physical-sensory facts. Then one may, if not yet advanced far in higher moral maturity, be inclined, with the intention of making what is to be communicated credible or convincing, to resort to frivolous means, for example by quoting statistics that cite millions of deaths caused by vaccination.

It is almost always the case that events, which appear as facts through extrasensory vision or research in the spiritual world, only appear on the physical plane with a certain time delay. One should not, however, feel pressured to resort to dishonest sources in the opinion that they would make the actual message more credible.

In the case of vaccinations against Sars-CoV-2, it may be that some people – not because of a basic interest in mysterious stories and interpretations (it should be noted in passing by the way, that today the more unspectacular of two variants of the interpretation of an event is usually the correct one), but in a kind of semi-consciousness or "clair-feeling," come to a certain conviction, the actual essence of which, however, they are neither able to clearly name nor to confirm by what is taking place in the physical domain, simply because what was perceived indistinctly at the spiritual level has not yet occurred on the physical-sensory level. For example, it may be that someone foresees through a kind of semi-consciousness what was the result of my spiritual contemplation as the Black Lodges' plan concerning vaccinations, but is not able to grasp it correctly as the plan which has not yet been realized at all. So that person cannot find the events expected by him on the physical domain (like, for example, the hundred-thousand-fold, million-fold deaths of people caused by vaccination). But he is so strongly convinced of his "finding," that he invents groundless "evidence" with which he seeks to substantiate it. But one must not, not even with passion for the spreading of truth, resort to the use of untruths because of spiritual and psychical immaturity!

In addition, I would like to note that in the case of the vaccinations now under discussion, I consider it impossible that they will cause a greater number of deaths *in the future*. And that *"mass"* deaths are occurring today due to vaccinations, as is being increasingly spread around from anthroposophical circles, is factually and simply incorrect. One can make such assertions either because of a seriously unhealthy psychical-spiritual constitution causing him to actually believe unreal things to be real, and therefore live in an world of illusionary thoughts, or because, due to moral immaturity – or whatever other motives may be involved, he is lying.

And indeed these observations on a sensory level, namely that *no* mass deaths have been caused by vaccination, also conclusively agree with my extrasensory investigations made already before the vaccinations were beginning to be used. In this respect, I now come back to the previously mentioned perfidious plan of the Black Lodges regarding vaccinations:

Thus, the current mRNA vaccination against the Sars-CoV-2 virus is a kind of Trojan horse – not a Trojan horse in terms of what it injects into the physical body of man, but what it injects into his soul. According to the plan of the Black Lodges, the harmless vaccination against Sars-CoV-2 is meant to make humanity have confidence in this kind of therapeutic treatment. For what they strive for is the manipulation of human DNA, because they want to procure power and other advantages by carving into the karmic plan, which is embedded in the DNA in respect to the physiological characteristics of the individual human being, meaning that it is present in the physical-material domain in the form of the DNA. The intent is to instill in humanity – through this vaccination, which promises a return to life as it was "before

Corona" – confidence in the harmlessness of this approach by vaccination. According to the corresponding

Black Lodges' plans, people are made to believe that: science, conventional medicine and pharmaceutical companies all care about my well-being, they make sure that I am protected from illness and death by vaccinations and applicable medications which, because of their fantastic new technology or active ingredients, cause no side effects, or hardly any, so that I can return to the lifestyle I had before.

It is already being claimed that diseases such as cancer or multiple sclerosis could be prevented in the future on the basis of such vaccinations as the mRNA or DNA. It may sound tempting, and it could put whoever is opposed to such "therapy" in a dim light. But it should be clear to anyone familiar with anthroposophy that the artificial "eradication" of illnesses brings with it the serious problem of having therewith destroyed an important path which the I chooses for fulfilling its karmic obligations, also an opportunity of an awakening towards spiritual reality. So other ways must be found by the extrasensory human being, who finally descends in order to incarnate, to achieve independent and conscious higher knowledge and thereby actual freedom, independence from any god, be it good or evil, so that he is able to reach a goal, namely spirit-knowledge and to voluntarily join the covenant with the "good God." However,

THE CORONAVIRUS PANDEMIC II

paths such as an illness (not contaminated by Soratic impulses) are eliminated by such measures. This is the door through which humanity is tempted to enter by the will of the Black Lodges. And if it does pass through, if it does not recognize vaccination against Sars-CoV-2 as a means chosen by the Black Lodges to awaken unjustified confidence in the "therapies" to follow in the future, then humanity will not only deprive itself of many ways by which individual karma can be fulfilled, but it also threatens to be led into captivity by means of the *prenatal* manipulation of the physical seed of man, by those circles which work against the good-divine world plan for the higher development of humanity.

To conclude this essay, I will risk speaking about a very unconventional and quite precarious measure, which is open to the student of the spirit who is threatened today by an infection with Sars-CoV-2, in order to procure the *time* needed for higher development in order to defend himself against the accusatory attacks by the counter-spiritual powers.

Whoever has read more closely Rudolf Steiner's three lectures in Dornach from November 1917, which are compiled under the title "The Right and Wrong Uses of Esoteric Knowledge," might have "stumbled" over a statement by Rudolf Steiner which gives cause for reflection in a special direction; the statement that in the present, fifth post-Atlantean age, humanity can develop *"by the incorporation of the forces of evil in the good sense"* (GA 178) to great spiritual ability, by which, as it were, evil can be transformed into good.

But I don't necessarily want to appeal to that statement. For it refers to those people who will have come to a real knowledge of Christ in the sense of Paul. But this does not yet apply to every human being who, however, with serious effort has already engaged in the soul-spiritual training path. I would like to refer instead – although I believe that Rudolf Steiner's statement may well refer to the possibility now to be mentioned – to another source, namely to the evangelist Matthew, who reproduces the words of Jesus Christ:

"See, I am sending you out like sheep into the midst of wolves; so be wise as serpents and innocent as doves."

(Matthew 10,16)

The conscientious spiritual student has – according to what results from my extrasensory and sensory observation – the opportunity to gain time by means of a vaccination against the coronavirus for the intensive development and purifying of his soul on the path of training, as it is outlined in the book *"How to gain knowledge of the higher worlds."* In a certain sense evil – or planned evil – can be beaten with its own weapons by the provisional protection that comes through vaccination which protects the anthroposophical spiritual student, or any human being from being robbed, by the consequences of a Covid-19 infection, of the time needed for their seriously desired and sought for spiritual development. Evil can be transformed into good *if* they actually use the time made available to them to do this work with unbridled earnestness, that is, to work spiritually on the development of the soul unperturbed by the Soratic attack. For in this way alone the means can grow for them, at the latest in the next incarnation, to help humanity and world existence to achieve its proper calling and mission, as able helpers of the good-divine Spirit, equipped with new abilities, not as "servants" but as "friends" of Christ. (Jn 15:12-15)

If the spiritual student obtains this advantage, this benefit, because of the vaccination, he or she has the absolute *obligation* to concentrate on this path of inner soul maturity with the utmost consistency – as does every other person. It's really not asking too much! For they are exercises that everyone can practice – if they really want to and are able to realize the extreme seriousness of the situation. But they must not want to acquire this benefit for their own sakes alone, but to acquire it with the moral attitude that they does so in order to mature spiritually in such a way that they are able to render a truly effective service to the world, and to human development as a whole, in the future!

It should be noted, however, that vaccination as such is not the solution to the problem; this should also have been clear from what was stated in Volume I. There is neither a guarantee of complete protection from an infection (even if in principle the encounter with the virus after a vaccination is mild, because then, due to the encounter not being with the harmful whole virus as previously, but only with the "sheath" of the virus, which has not yet fully awakened to the vegetative processes of the physical body, the I can become effective again in the old way from the extrasensory periphery) nor will this kind of vaccination work permanently and against all mutations of the Sars-CoV-2 virus, which will still develop if the vaccinations are utilized without any spiritual consciousness work being undertaken by humanity. If humanity does not now deign to acknowledge the threefold spiritual nature of the one Logos, if it does not seek its moral ideals at the level of living reality, then the positive effects of the vaccination will peter out. Then it becomes more like a boomerang, which loops back at us and – just as *not* vaccinating (and by this we see what a tricky situation we've got ourselves involved in) – leads to ever more dangerous variants of the virus, which finally achieve what the opposing sub-sensory spiritual force intended to achieve by the virus. Vaccinations will then foster the mutation and increasing resistance of the viruses, and long-term symptoms may then come after infection that have not previously appeared or have not appeared to the extent expected. And finally an awakening to spiritual realities, which include first and foremost the recognition of the human being as a pure spirit, as well as knowledge of the so-called *deed* of Christ for humanity. If this does not happen, the germination of pathogens will occur compared to which the destructive potential of the Sars-CoV-2 virus becomes almost unremarkable.

To the question of vaccination, the person who is burning for knowing the living spirit can actually only ask himself whether he decides for "plague or cholera" or – perhaps not quite so drastically – for plague or a sprained ankle. Because at some point he *will* come into contact with the Sars-CoV-2 virus. The fact that humans must deal with the viral wrapper (or sheath) protein in the course of a vaccination is a fact. I will have something to say elsewhere in detail, at a later date, about what this means. But the controversy about what constitutes the totality of the virus (there can be no question of a total "organism," as already stated in Volume I) is, from a spiritual standpoint, a completely different dimension.

And at present we may still assume that an infection with Sars- CoV-2 after vaccination does not usually lead to (physical and spiritual) long-term consequences, as it does in the case of an infection without prior vaccination.

The spiritual student must consider whether he would rather risk meeting the opponent of the I on the level of his physical body, almost unarmed, and accept the long arm of this opponent of the I in his etheric, astral and I organism, with its devastating effects and, moreover, risk being jointly responsible for the infection of other people; or whether by obtaining some protection he runs the risk, as a vaccinated person, of giving the wrong impression to his spiritually ignorant surroundings, namely the impression that there is a security which is easy to obtain without any effort of his own. For he runs this risk if he is perceived in his circle only as being vaccinated, but not as a living example of someone who identifies with the spirit. And he must ask himself whether he even wants to risk being directly responsible for the emergence of even worse scenarios, with the most serious consequences, being vaccinated and simultaneously neglecting the necessary psychical self-education. (Those who are not vaccinated must of course ask themselves the same questions.) As far as my insight tells me, the second option can still lead to something positive, because the conditions for its favorable outcome can certainly be fulfilled by people who are seriously concerned about the living spirit, or even a spiritual student. It would require, however, a certain number of human souls, for it is a karmic event happening to humanity as a whole.

We must realize that there is no way out of this situation completely untouched. That is why a "*spirituel Ratio*" and a "spiritual rationality" are needed. And this does not only mean choosing to be vaccinated in order to comply with Christ's instruction to be "wise" "like serpents," but at the same time to strive for that moral purity in one's own soul, for which the image of the dove was chosen, which in Christian iconography appears as God's messenger, as the Holy Spirit.

Humanity today must get around to basing its opinions and actions on something other than sensory-intellectual ratio – "*What must we do to perform the works of God?*" Christ's answer to this is, "*This is the work of God, that you believe in him whom he has sent.*" (John 6:28-29)

Why is faith in Christ – which today in the age of the consciousness soul expresses willingness to know Christ – necessary to do good works? It is necessary because Christ is the spirit of *truth*. In our thinking we must seek the connection to truth. We must give up lying, but also speculation, half-truths, hyper-rationality, intellectual as well as the unworldly, Luciferic, irrational confusion of our minds. This is achievable through the path of selflessness, on which Christ preceded us as an example. The creative "Word," which was in the beginning and from which the world came forth, lives in the truth, which it proclaimed itself. Whoever looks to the representative of humanity, whoever hears his voice, does not find it difficult to bear the cross of renunciation of personal advantage, and will find the narrow but sure way of the middle. The connection with Christ lifts the person over his weaknesses and makes him a helper on the great work of humanity's development – What are we waiting for?

Appendix

The parable of the unjust steward according to Luke 16, 1-9

He also said to His disciples:

There was a certain rich man who had a steward, and an accusation was brought to him that this man was wasting his goods. So he called him and said to him, What is this I hear about you? Give an account of your stewardship, for you can no longer be steward.

Then the steward said to himself, What shall I do? For my master is taking the stewardship away from me. I cannot dig; I am ashamed to beg. I have resolved what to do, that when I am put out of the stewardship, they may receive me into their houses.

So he called every one of his master's debtors to him, and said to the first, 'How much do you owe my master?' And he said, A hundred measures of oil. So he said to him, Take your bill, and sit down quickly and write fifty. Then he said to another, And how much do you owe? So he said, A hundred measures of wheat. And he said to him, Take your bill, and write eighty.

So the master commended the unjust steward because he had dealt shrewdly. For the sons of this world are more shrewd in their generation than the sons of light.

And I say to you, make friends with the unrighteous mammon, that when you fail, they may receive you into an everlasting home.

This parable is certainly somewhat "awkward," because it is difficult to reconcile these words of Christ with the other virtues known as "Christian."

It may also be because nowadays we are no longer familiar with the kind of Pharisaic-Sadducee sophistry of those times, whereby one often spoke in a roundabout way, so to speak. The master obviously resorted to it here for his purposes. I mean that one may understand this passage basically quite "simply" and interpret it more or less as follows:

Obviously this parable is not about the teaching of economics, but – as written – it is a *parable*, which is why it is not about earthly, but about spiritual goods.

The preceding parables (in Luke 15) all refer to the soul--spiritual return from the diaspora of aberration to the divine-spiritual home based of the insight of the person concerned.

For even though in the first parable (unlike in the two that follow) it is the shepherd who brings back his sheep, the occasion for this parable was that the "tax collectors and sinners" "continually drew near" to the Lord, that is, expressed a longing of their own accord for his instruction and help, whereupon the scribes criticized His dealings with them. It is true that the parable of the unjust steward is addressed "also" to the disciples, as it says, but the scribes are still present, and before their eyes and ears Christ advises the disciples what they should think of the conduct of these scribes, how they should classify it, evaluate it. Then He turns again to the

Pharisees with the clear words: "*It is you who make yourselves appear righteous before men, but God knows your hearts ...*" (Luke 16:15)

In this overall context, then, the parable of the unjust steward is given, and one may become aware that in terms of content and style, it is similar to the parables in Matthew ("*But the kingdom of heaven is like ...*" or the parable of the owner of the vineyard).

With the example of the unjust scribes, the disciples were to learn something about how to handle the spiritual gifts given to them by God. For it is they, after all, who will be sent out to proclaim the Gospel, the New Covenant of God, to the peoples in all the world. Since the Lord had chosen them to be His apostles, because they had known Him and had therefore been given to Him by the Father (Jn 17, Farewell Prayer) – according to the Prologue, that is, as "children of God" "who received Him" – it was indisputable that these Twelve were initially ahead of their human brethren in the knowledge of Christ and the aims of the New Covenant. They had been given special gifts, but at the same time this brought with it equally great responsibilities. (Attention is already drawn to this fact in the main text).

"To whom much is entrusted, more will be required," Luke 12, 48

But before the disciples (uneducated in the study of the Scriptures, but whose hearts were directly trained by Jesus Christ) were entrusted with the administration of the Word, an administration that had been taken over by the scribes – a notoriously degenerate connection to the tradition of the Old Covenant, when spiritual matters were still in the hands of a designated group, which was able to receive Yahweh's instructions instead of the people, and was thus kept "pure" as a priestly lineage through bloodlines. As initiates, this group administered a knowledge that was withheld from the others.

This was to fundamentally change with the establishment of the New Covenant. How else should we understand the words: *"Nothing is covered up that will not be uncovered, and nothing hidden that will not become known. What I say to you in the dark, tell in the light, and what you hear whispered, proclaim from the housetops."* (Matthew 10-26,27) or *"No one after lighting a lamp hides it in a jar or puts it under a bed, but puts it on a lampstand, so those who enter may see the light. For nothing is hidden that will not be revealed ..."* (Luke 8,16 f) Each individual human being, through the sacrificial death of Christ, should be lent the tools to be able as an individual to become, as it were, a "priest" himself one day through his faith in Christ, a responsible person in the sense of the Holy Spirit, or an initiate in the Pauline sense with direct knowledge of the reality of the Risen One. In the future, knowledge of the mystery-secrets should no longer be kept for one alone, but in so far as he or she may know more than others, they are obliged to share it with the others in a responsible way. In other words, the disciples were not to imitate the scribes, who watched over the divine teaching, claimed its sovereignty of interpretation for themselves alone and judged others according to their discretion.

Against this background, the *"rich man"* in the parable of the unjust *steward* seems to be God himself (his wealth is the "kingdom of heaven," divine wisdom and love), and the "steward" of his property is the one who is chosen to have a certain insight into or participation in this property, which in return obliges him to manage it in a right way. The way in which the steward "squanders" the master's "property" however, consists in using the spiritual goods entrusted to him for himself alone, that is, in misusing them and, moreover, making others dependent by demanding interest and keeping it for himself.

Then, when the steward is admonished by his master, he devises a clever bargain to buy himself free by giving away the master's goods (in form of the forgiven debt). And this is what the master praises in response!

What are the disciples (those who want to follow Christ) to learn from this?

Toward those to whom they are sent out, they should deal in the same way with the gifts given to them as the steward deals with the rich master's property toward the indebted trading partners – but for opposite motives. ("*For the sons of this world are wiser in their generation than the sons of light.*") In this parable, the unjust Mammon stands for the keeping for yourself of spiritual goods, which are actually entrusted to you for the purpose of increasing them by giving them away ("... I have appointed you to go and bear fruit, and that your fruit will last, so that the Father may give you whatever you ask him in my name," John 15, 16, see also the parable of the entrusted talents. Luke 19, 11 ff and Matthew 25, 14 ff) If the unjust steward's behavior is applied to the handling of spiritual gifts, the Gospel will spread and the apostles and all the witnesses to the reality of Christ will bear "fruit." By giving away the Lord's spiritual property, it is increased among the people.

"Make friends with the unrighteous mammon, that when you fail, they may receive you into an everlasting home."

If we apply the "model" of the unjust steward to the spiritual, we are "wise" but "without falsehood," and we will make friends both among the people, to whom we will give the possessions (which we have wrongfully kept for ourselves), and at the same time make friends with the angels, who will one day admit us to their dwellings in return.

The present passage can be understood in this sense. It fits with a sentence which is taken from a lecture by Rudolf Steiner in *"Background to the Gospel of Mark,"* where it is written as a concluding remark. Whoever is familiar with the meaning of the gospel passage touched on here will perhaps also see this connection: *"But what lies dormant in the future can come to life if there are enough people who know that knowledge is a duty, because we may not return our souls to* the world-spirit undeveloped; for then we will have taken something from the world-spirit itself which it has incorporated into us." (GA 124)

About the Author

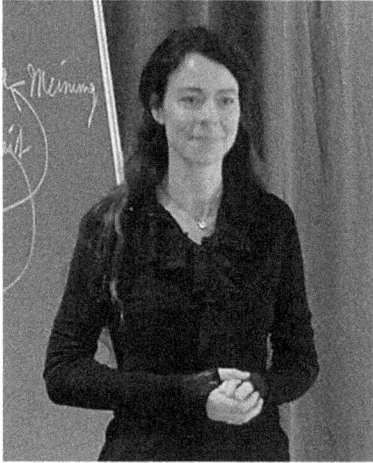

JUDITH VON HALLE was born 1972 in Berlin. She is an architect by profession and has worked as such. She has felt herself to be especially bound to Christ since childhood. She encountered anthroposophy in 1997 and worked part time for the German Anthroposophical Society until 2005. From 2001 till 2003 she gave lectures in the Rudolf Steiner House about esoteric Judaism and the Apocalypse of St. John.

During Easter 2004 the stigmata of Christ appeared on her. Since that happened she has only been able to consume water – that is, no solid nourishment. She gives lectures and writes books that are mostly, but not exclusively concerned with Christology, whereby she adheres to Rudolf Steiner's work on the same subject.

As is true with other stigmata cases, Judith von Halle can "see" the events during the life of Jesus. She speaks of "time travel". As of now she has written 18 books. The series "Contributions towards an Understanding of the Christ event" contain descriptions from her time travels.

Judith and her husband Carl-August live in Berlin, but travel to Dornach often.

www.ingramcontent.com/pod-product-compliance
Lightning Source LLC
Chambersburg PA
CBHW070122030426

42335CB00016B/2240